Andrea ♔ **W9-BEK-565**

VOICES THAT CARE

Also by Neal Hitchens:

Fifty Things You Can Do About AIDS

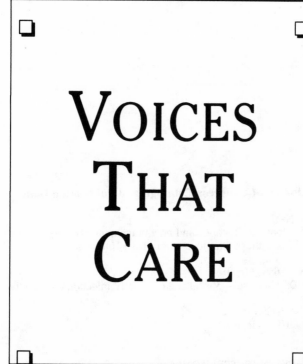

VOICES THAT CARE

Stories and Encouragements
for People with AIDS/HIV
and Those Who Love Them

NEAL HITCHENS

LOWELL HOUSE
LOS ANGELES
CONTEMPORARY BOOKS
CHICAGO

Library of Congress Cataloging-in-Publication Data

Hitchens, Neal.
    Voices that care : stories and encouragements for people with
AIDS/HIV and those who love them / Neal Hitchens.
        p.   cm.
    ISBN 1-56565-006-9
    1. AIDS (Disease)—Miscellanea.   2. HIV infections—Miscellanea.
I. Title.
RC607.A26H553   1992
362.1′969792—dc20

92-13920
CIP

Requests for such permissions should be addressed to:
Lowell House
2029 Century Park East, Suite 3290
Los Angeles, CA 90067

PUBLISHER: Jack Artenstein
EXECUTIVE VICE-PRESIDENT: Nick Clemente
VICE-PRESIDENT/EDITOR-IN-CHIEF: Janice Gallagher
DESIGN: Stanley S. Drate/Folio Graphics, Inc.

Manufactured in the United States of America

10   9   8   7   6   5   4   3   2   1

TO
Christopher Esposito
for opening my heart;

TO
Randall Riese
for opening my mind.

We're each handed an empty sketch pad, and a box of Crayolas, and we're told to draw. What we choose to put on that paper, however, is up to us.

—RANDALL RIESE

CONTENTS

ACKNOWLEDGMENTS

For their inspiration, support, and belief in me: Christopher Esposito, Mark Goins, Sydney and Donald Hitchens, Randall Riese.

For her belief in this project from its inception, and for her truly fine editorial contributions: Janice Gallagher.

For their humanity: the many people who shared with me their personal stories. I would have liked to have included them all.

And for their various and much appreciated contributions to this work, the individuals and organizations listed below:

AIDS Project Los Angeles
Alison Arngrim
Wendy Arnold
Being Alive
Howard Bragman
Lisa Brown
Steve Burns
Brad Cafarelli
The Center
Century City Hospital,
    Special Care Unit
Rob Clauson
Matt DeHaven
Roger Duncan
Fletcher Foster
Mark Gifford
John Grasso

Dr. Ralph Hansen
Pat Harvey
Peter Hoffman
Alan Hymowitz
Sally Jue
Kim Kiosow
Project Angel Food
Project Open Hand
Dina Rosen
Steve Sanders
Shanti
Kim Swann
Tuesday's Child
Rhonda Tuman
Robert Waldron
Freddie Weber
Dr. Peter Wolfe

◻ Voices That Carry ◻

The numbers, certainly, are staggering. One in every 100 men in the United States is infected with the HIV virus. Every 13 minutes, another person in this country is infected. Women are being infected at an alarming rate and represent the fastest rising so-called risk group. And yet, the response from the federal government has been woefully disproportionate to the tragedy. Members of the entertainment industry, however, as well as certain other public figures, have utilized their celebrity to promote messages of AIDS education, funding for research, and compassion.

In developing this book, dozens of celebrities were contacted and asked one simple question: "If you could say something to someone with AIDS, what would you say?"

◻

I was a member of my high school's marching band. During football games, out on the field, we would play "We Will Rock You," the song by Queen, because it always pumped up the team as well as the audience. Even though we used to put as much energy as possible into performing that single, nothing compared to Freddie Mercury and Queen's version. When I was a young wannabe musician, Mercury was one of my idols. His death, combined with the passing of fashion designer Willi Smith, impacted my life, as I became aware of the fact that AIDS has taken some of my heroes.

My father was a powerful and knowledgeable Baptist preacher. The things he taught me still hold true today, with one exception: He said that bad things don't happen to good people. My dad never knew about AIDS because he passed away in the mid-'70s, before the country became aware of this killer. A very bad thing has happened to many, many good people. I hope that they know they have nothing to be ashamed of. If my father was alive now, I'm sure his teachings would change, to encourage all of us to unite and fight this disease together.

—ARSENIO HALL

❏

I will still do fund-raising work for AMFAR [American Foundation for AIDS Research], but they are involved in the medical side of AIDS, which is great. But I've seen so many people suffering from AIDS that I want to be more personally involved with them. I want to help those who are suffering *now.*

What would I say to people with AIDS?

Honey, hang in there. We will win, we will win!

—ELIZABETH TAYLOR

❏

2

I became involved in AIDS because it was in front of me: Many people I knew were HIV-positive. It was clear to me how much of a difference human compassion can make. I don't think AIDS is any different than any other human heartbreak. But no human heartbreak is as hard to endure when someone puts their arms around you and is there for you and truly cares.

—*MARIANNE WILLIAMSON*

❏

The AIDS crisis. I think it ought to be at the top of the national health-care agenda. The president barely mentions it. You've got a million and a half people dying of AIDS; you've got good research projects that are not being funded; you've got people who, while we're waiting for one or the other of these health-care plans, can't get covered. They're suffering, and no other country, at least developed country, would let that happen. I think the president's got to stand up and say, "Look, we've got a plague on our hands. We've got to talk about it—how it's transmitted. We've got to warn people, and we've got to pay the money so that we don't abandon people who are suffering and dying in every community in America.

—*JERRY BROWN*
former California governor and
1992 presidential candidate

❏

I believe God is always there with us in our hearts and our minds. He may come to us in the shape of many things, a smile, a sunrise, a kind word, or an understanding look. He may come to

3

us disguised as a hilarious joke or the ability to laugh at ourselves and our situation in our most desperate hours.

—*CHER*

❏

I'm a science nut. And I started reading these blurbs of these isolated cases of strange immune deficiencies. I was very interested because it was something new out there that nobody seemed to be paying any attention to. That was in 1980, 1981, before there were fund-raisers, before it even had a name. People really didn't pay attention until that summer Rock Hudson got sick. Suddenly, we'd be driving to a location in the morning for "Falcon Crest," and I'd be doing a symposium on AIDS all the way to the location. And all the way back, people were saying, "Oh, dear, that was *the thing* you were talking about, Morgan." And all of a sudden, they started asking all these questions. That summer I really realized that there was a place for me to do something here.

It's kind of a strange thing, because in L.A., when you come out here, you are hounded by these public-relations people who all want you to do charity work, things that make you look like a good person. And they'll pick some nice, innocuous charity for you to do. But if you picked something like AIDS or abortion rights, which are the things I work on, people say, "You don't have to do that. No, no, no."

I've seen so many of my friends make great use of the time they have left. To them, all I can say is: "What do you need? What do you want? Can I help? Do you need to cry? Do you need to talk? Do you want to go to a movie?" Just anything I can do to make their life as normal, fun, and free of worry as possible.

That's why I'm here.

And I would say what my mother in Texas used to tell me when I'd get in a really bad way as a kid: "Just don't let the bastards get you down."

—*MORGAN FAIRCHILD*

❏

My love of my mother was the true discovery, for me, of eternal love. When she left us, it was then I knew we would only be temporarily separated, because love clings and becomes a part of you, gives you strength, and assures you that you will never be alone. Having learned this, I have been able to apply this to my many losses due to this dreadful disease, AIDS. The key is to *love* while we are here, and that will be our comfort for the short time we are separated. *They* would not like our being anything less than what they loved and knew. We carry on, not only for ourselves but for them. I do feel that I am being watched over, and I like it.

—*CHITA RIVERA*

❏

It's so wild now. . . . Growing up is so hard for kids. Kids look up to me because they can relate to me. They see me and they say that "yeah, he's had sex," you know? So I'm like saying to them, "Hey, buddy, before sliding in the shaft, Trojan the wood!"

—*PAULY SHORE*

❏

I think I'm involved with the fight against AIDS because at this particular time, I think it's perhaps the single most important health issue on a global scale. I've lost some very close and dear friends. Aside from the personal losses, it's afforded me a wonderful and rare opportunity to be a part of other people's lives. I think to lend dignity to someone's life, no matter what their situation, is one of the only real important things we can do for each other.

—*ARLO GUTHRIE*

❑

I would say that I cannot presume to know what your individual experience is, but whatever it is, I can understand and accept it. You must have whatever feelings you have, and you deserve to be supported in dealing with them and working your own way through them.

Neither I nor my life can ever be the same since the onslaught of AIDS. I genuinely feel that in spite of testing HIV-negative, I, like everyone else in the world, am "a person living with AIDS." In the '60s I listened to rhetoric about how "we are all one," and I agreed with it. But now it is so much more real to me. I see AIDS striking my friends and it truly feels like *I* have been struck. I see the government failing to respond proportionately to the level of crisis and it feels like they are underestimating the magnitude of *my* problem.

Whenever I look at it, I see that it would have been possible for the world to discover its unity through hunger or cancer or diabetes or MS or whatever (and many individuals have!), but my prayer is that *everyone* will come out of this experience with a very different

6

point of view—that as a society we will never, ever again think that something is happening to *"them."*

—JUDITH LIGHT

❏

First off, I can never, ever feel exactly what someone with AIDS is going through. But I do believe in laughter. There's an old saying: "Laugh in the face of death." Well, I think it needs to be revised to "Laugh in the face of life." Laughter inspires longevity.

—JAY THOMAS

❏

Hope and strength and friends . . . with these we *will* make it. Love to all.

—LIZA MINNELLI

❏

What would I say to a friend of mine who had AIDS?

Any friend of mine would know that I love them no matter what. I would try to help them live with the attitude that although they have AIDS, *it* doesn't have *them.*

And last, I would pray for them to know that God's love for them was all-merciful and eternal.

—DOLLY PARTON

❏

My spirits are lifted and I am inspired because William is *alive*—with every Christmas wreath, with every holiday bow, with every changing season and its flowers. And it reminds my heart that he is never truly gone. His gift and artistry live on, both seasonal and eternal, with every bloom.

—JOAN VAN ARK
in honor of her friend,
floral designer William Carl Alspaugh

❏

I've lost dear friends to AIDS, and it seems very sad that young and talented people have to go. I went to a lecture recently and there were a lot of myths about AIDS. I would encourage everybody to be as educated as possible about it.

I've met a lot of people with AIDS, and I've hugged and kissed them, but it makes you feel helpless that you can't do something to help them.

I've seen young people smoking [cigarettes] and they think that they're invincible, and you can see the same young people not caring about sexual protection. They think that it wouldn't happen to them. I would tell them to be very, very careful and *not* to think they are invincible.

What would I say to people with AIDS?

I understand that if you have a clean, healthy life-style, if you get your rest and eat healthily, and if you have a positive attitude, you can maybe prolong your life. And I see also that people get despondent and can give up. And as with anything, the attitude is obviously very important.

In [her teachings based on] *A Course in Miracles,* Marianne

8

Williamson reminds us that we all have a mind that is very powerful. And I believe that. I do.

—DOM DeLUISE

❑

I've lost too many precious people. I've seen them too lonely and too ostracized and go too unheeded. I'd say that the way AIDS has impacted my life, for the most part, is that it has instilled a lot of anger in me; anger at society's denial of this disease, especially at the beginning, and anger at the ostracism of people who are gay.

I would also say that everything that happens to us happens for a reason. There is a lesson we're learning in all of this. We're going to grow through it, and it's going to be even more beautiful and more knowledgeable for the next world.

—HEATHER THOMAS

❑

When I have felt the most terrified and lost in my life, the only true solace that will ever quiet my aching heart is my connection with God. I have only to ask God to hold me in His loving arms and protect me from my fear, and eventually I will get still. And in that stillness I know that I will be taken care of every moment. And in that very moment I am fine.

I never know what trials life will bring me, but I have a faith that even when things seem truly hopeless, I will be given what I need.

—LESLEY ANN WARREN

❑

A deadly disease doesn't strike home until someone close to you gets it, but, like a black cloud on the horizon, none of us can ignore the facts, the numbers, and the threat of the deadly HIV virus. It's a problem for all of us.

—LEE GREENWOOD

❑

My dear friend Fern Fields passed this beautiful story on to me. Its poignant message touched me. I hope you like it too.

As the old man walked the beach at dawn, he noticed a young woman ahead of him picking up starfish and flinging them into the sea. Finally catching up with the youth, he asked her why she was doing this. The answer was that the stranded starfish would die if left until the morning sun.

"But the beach goes on for miles, and there are millions of starfish," countered the old man. "How can your effort make any difference?"

The young woman looked at the starfish in her hand and threw it safely into the waves. "It makes a difference to this one," she said.

Love and laughter . . .

—ESTELLE GETTY

❑

Oh, God, I've had so many friends who have died of AIDS.

I've spent my entire adult life on television, starting in 1972 with "Maude." In between television shows I had a very close friend, the friend I saw day-to-day, who was dying of AIDS. He was in and out of the Veterans Hospital in Westwood, close to where I live, and I found myself going there daily whenever he was hospitalized. From my own personal experience with friends who have suffered from AIDS, I had very little hope. AIDS isn't pretty. I also believe in death with dignity. And I believe that when the shit hits the fan, if you'll pardon the expression, one should have the option of deciding one's own fate of ending one's own life if things get to be too painful and horrible. It's our right.

I think it is horrendous that it has come to *this*. This disease has been killing the gay community for the past 10 years, and nobody would listen.

Before Magic [Johnson] came out, I had no hope for a cure in the near future. But now I really do have hope. Magic's coming out has given me hope that money will now be spent to find a cure. Now there *is* hope, because AIDS will be taken seriously. Until Magic, unless people were directly involved with someone who had AIDS, they really didn't care. Certainly George Bush and his administration were not taking it seriously, and I think now that has all changed. Now the public feels they have to *do* something. I feel that now money will be spent and that we *will* find a cure.

—*BEA ARTHUR*

❏

Never, ever, ever, ever, ever, ever, ever, ever, ever, ever give up hope.

We will win. We will win in the end.

—*JOAN RIVERS*

11

I don't care what God you pray to. It doesn't matter what religion you are. You don't have to pray to Jesus if you don't want to. I mean, I'm Jewish, you know? But what it comes down to is prayer. There is a God up there. I've been praying, and things have been happening. Miracles, you know? He doesn't come down here and say, "Here I am," but He sends people into my life who are spiritual and helpful. Maybe you can't take away all of the pain. But if you have peace of mind, the pain doesn't hurt so much. It doesn't matter as much. Do you hear me?

—ALI GERTZ
Ali Gertz died of AIDS in August 1992.
She was the subject of a 1992 made-for-
television movie. She was 26 years old.

❏

I want a world where there is no closet. I sat in the hospital room with Ryan White and the respirator and saw the horrible close-up look at the death of a young boy. I'll never forget it. I think the slogan "Silence Equals Death" has finally seeped into the American consciousness.

I'm feeling depressed and am appalled by my own church's legitimization of homophobia. I think the church's continued preachments which prohibit Catholics' use of condoms are irresponsible. Wake up!

—PHIL DONAHUE

12

ONE VOICE

*I*t was August 31, 1990, when the caller came knocking at my front door. The pounding was rude, incessant. It wouldn't go away. It wasn't Avon calling; it was AIDS. My life partner of seven years, Christopher Esposito, was rushed to the hospital in a coma. "AIDS," they said. "Six months," they said. I clasped my hands over my ears, but the message penetrated through. Death. Destruction. Gloom. Doom. I screamed the loudest scream I ever heard in my life. It emerged from my gut and built up momentum as it raced to my heart, to the lump in my throat, to my mouth. But no sound passed my lips as the scream echoed through my brain. I've always had a problem with expressing my fears and feelings, and so I swallowed my voice. I swallowed my pain.

I knew that I had to get tested. I should've been tested years before, but I hid, foolishly, behind that tired (and dangerous) cliché, "It can't happen to me." Yeah, right. I walked into the doctor's office alone. I was the last patient of the day. Two weeks later I returned to get my results. The office was cold, stark, garishly lit. There was no "hello." There was no "how are you?" Just a nurse with a death sentence. "Mr. Hitchens," she said, "your test came back positive."

I was numb. Alone. Chris was still in the hospital. I wanted to take a bath. I called my best friend, Randall. He was obviously, audibly upset. He expressed his feelings and asked me about mine. But at that point, I didn't know how or what I felt, or how to express it if I did.

In the succeeding weeks, as the news settled into my consciousness, I made a vow to myself. I was going to learn everything I could about this virus that I had. I was going to help others who were sick. I was going to volunteer my time to the local AIDS service organizations. I was going to be Chris's primary caregiver, while continuing to work my full-time job. And I was going to do it all with a smile and without telling others about my own status. You know the scene in *Gypsy* when Rosalind Russell tells Natalie Wood to get on the stage and become a stripper? A look of resignation and acceptance comes over Natalie's face. A look that says, "OK. You want me to be a stripper? I'm going to be the best damn stripper you've ever seen!" Well, I was going to be the best damn HIV-positive person that anyone had ever seen.

How has AIDS changed me? Growing up in Georgetown, Delaware, I couldn't wait to move to the big city. I wanted to be famous. I wanted to prove to everybody that I was somebody. Over the last two years, AIDS has taught me that *everybody* is somebody, and you don't have to prove anything to anybody but yourself. Growing up in Georgetown, I wanted to see the world. Today, more and more, I long to move back home.

I think I've learned that I don't have to be a perfect Boy Scout. When I look into the mirror I see a boy who wanted it all and is probably going to have to settle for less. But that's OK. I see a boy who is trying hard to be John Wayne brave but who doesn't always succeed. And that's OK. And over my shoulder in the mirror I always, always see Randall.

I've learned that being HIV-positive is not necessarily a death sentence.

Perhaps most important, I've learned how to share my feelings. I used to feel that the people I loved knew it—sort of a quiet understanding—and it didn't need to be expressed. Not anymore. Just say it. It's better than AZT. It's better than DDI [Dideoxyinosine]. It's better than Zovirax, and without the toxicity. Christopher, I love you. Randall, I love you. Mark, I love you. Mom and Dad, I love you.

The knocking, by the way, has subsided. I've opened the front door and accepted AIDS into my living room. We're not friends by any means, but we've negotiated a truce of sorts. I still don't like him, this bully virus called HIV, but I've gotten to know him, and I've learned from him, and I'm no longer afraid of him. In fact, on a good day, I think of him as just a tenant, renting space in my body. He can be a bitch, and he can wreak havoc, but sometimes I have to remind him who's the landlord, who's the boss.

Voices That Care gives a voice to the tens of thousands of sons, daughters, mothers, fathers, grandchildren, and grandparents who are living and dying with AIDS. For this is no longer a disease of the so-called risk groups. Actually, it never was. It is a disease of families and friends.

There are frighteningly few defenses against the AIDS virus, but among the strongest is the will to love, live, and help one another. More than 1,000 people responded to the call of this book to share their stories with the hope that, by doing so, they will help untold thousands of others who might be going through a similar experience.

Voices That Care is not a medical or psychological text. Instead, it expresses simply and without affectation the poignant voices of those who have been fighting on the front lines of this disease:

15

those who have developed full-blown AIDS and are near death; those who have tested HIV-positive and are counting their tomorrows; those who have had lovers taken from their arms; and those who have had their children deteriorate before their eyes.

Why have I written this book? Because it's what *I* can do. Because I'm no longer willing to swallow my voice. Alone, I may be a whisper, but in unison with the nearly 100 other voices presented in these pages, I am a chorus.

—NEAL HITCHENS
Los Angeles, 1992

STORIES AND ENCOURAGEMENTS

I was diagnosed on a dark, cold night last winter. I knew I probably had *it*. I'd been sicker than usual. So had my best friends (I've lost 14, including my three best friends).

I hadn't lived as Mother Teresa. However, what I *didn't* expect was the subtle change in the way I now perceive and prioritize *everything* and *everyone*. So much just doesn't matter anymore. So much else is equally and simply priceless, such as friends (sick or well) and my own health.

Now, each day is a wonderful reprieve, each hour without aches and pains a bonus, and each doctor's office visit is either a routine prophylaxis or another crash course in symptoms, diagnoses, and a trip to the friendly pharmacy. Is each pimple KS [Kaposi's sarcoma]? Each cough PCP [pneumocystis carinii pneumonia]? Each bump some lymph-node trouble?

Am I angry? No! I played. I pay. I have no regrets! In my mirror I now see something new: a fighter and a survivor, willing to do anything to stay alive—as long as it is a quality life. I'm sympathetic to most of the goals of ACT-UP [AIDS Coalition to Unleash Power]; hopeful of a vaccine; overwhelmed by the loss of *sooooo* much talent, the size of The Quilt [an AIDS memorial in progress]; and

17

the hope that "chronic manageable lifetime illness" will kick in before I check out.

Life is still very good, has much to offer, even with my immune problems. The alternative is another memorial service, another loss. Fighters last longer. I'm a fighter, fighting for my life.

At a camp my parents sent my brother and me to when we were young, there was a sign hung in the dining room that read: WHEN YOU THINK YOU HAVE NOTHING TO BE THANKFUL FOR, BE THANKFUL FOR SOME OF THE THINGS YOU *DON'T* HAVE. This may sound morbid, but I have pictures of me with most of the friends I've lost to AIDS. I've had five-by-seven photos made that are up on my wall in a collage. It's a place of honor. It's really important for me to focus on them in my prayers. And yet that motto from camp keeps coming back when I think of the MAI [mycobacterium avium intracellulare], the KS, the toxoplasmosis, and some of the really awful things that some of my buddies have had and had to deal with. Boy, I don't have a problem in the world compared to what they went through. So I am grateful for the things that I *don't* have and don't have to deal with. At least not yet.

I'm not giving up. It may sound a little goofy, but I don't want to jump right on the medical prescription bandwagon. I've opted not to go on AZT or DDI at this time. I don't want to do that. I know it's pretty toxic stuff. I know that everything is a trade-off, but at this point I just don't want to put that stuff in my body. I am doing Zovirax, and I'm also eating bananas for neuropathy. But that's about it. For now, I'm doing OK. If I were to have another major episode of something, I would probably reconsider, but I think I have some time.

I've also joined Test Positive Aware, a support group here in Chicago that's been pretty significant to me. I very much like the

"Ask the Doctor" nights that they have about once every five weeks. The question-and-answer periods are incredibly informative, and I'm always asking questions. I also read a lot. I get *Project Informed, Data, New York Native,* and the TPA newsletter. I read the gay rags every week, not in a phobic way, but just because I want to be informed.

What do I miss most?

Having sex without rubbers. I really miss that.

What would I say to other people?

The most important thing is to listen to your body. That sounds awfully simplistic, probably, but I think it's the thing that has worked most for me and for a couple of my friends. It tells me when I need to eat. It tells me when I need to rest. I get really tired now. When my friend was here from out of town, I took a nap twice a day for 15 or 20 minutes. I just lay down and did nothing but listen to my body. It may sound like voodoo, but it really does work.

What was my childhood ambition?

I wanted to be a king and live in a castle. Also, when I was 10, I wrote something called "My Ambition." It was done on that old wide-line paper, and my penmanship was just horrible because I was just learning to write instead of print. Now, I have it up on my wall. Let me share it with you:

I want to be an animal doctor. I want to take care of sick animals. I want to take care of animals when their owners go away. When I retire, I want a parrot, a dog, a kitten, two goldfish, a monkey, and a canary.

I would like to live in a very big house.
I want two butlers, two maids. I want
a wife to share my life.

Well, I've changed some of that.

—*BILL HANSON*

☐ Bill Hanson, 47, is an administrative secretary. He was
diagnosed with pneumocystis and AIDS on December
14, 1990. As of this writing, he is still working, still
healthy, and still fighting.

The Wayland Flowers House is an AIDS residential hospice in Los Angeles. Charles Palmisano was a resident there for seven months before his death on September 17, 1991. At that time, Paul Hedge, hospice manager, found in Charles's personal belongings an introductory note and essay that had been written by Charles as he approached death. The administrative staff at Wayland Flowers has graciously allowed us to reprint them both below.

*E*ighteen years ago my assignment for English composition was a one-page essay. It was accepted by my professor only after three drafts and my grouching to the department chairman that I didn't have the time or interest to devote to the subject. Truthfully, I lacked the talent and insight to even begin. I seem to recall a D.

Yet, since school, I've often lain in bed at night in darkness, and thoughts form and flowingly crystallize—usually sharper, more lucid and lyrical than the attached.

I still know nothing about writing. But tonight, "The View from My Room" emerged. It's a gift I can now enjoy just for myself, and perhaps later it will touch someone else who may find it.

It may be too amateurish to share, but still I'm happy not to have the talent of a writer to burden my conscience.

This may be the paper my instructor was trying to get out of me.

The View from My Room

By Charles Palmisano

As I lie on my bed, gazing out of my window, the act of expressing my thoughts brings a new perspective and appreciation of the beauty beside me.

Straight ahead, to the right, and across the green grass lies a heavily foliaged patch of plant life native to our tightly grouped outpoint. Great, lofty flowers glow with yellows, golds, and rusts against the gray and drab that predominate in this world.

Plants are freely interspersed, their clumps bringing in bright and pale greens of illumination. They are energetic, healthy, life-affirming sights among the fading and aging shade trees. They are matched ideally and joyously to their surroundings.

Ahead of the thicket bloom bouquets of flowers, their colors astonishing. Looking out the window through the rectangular frame brings to mind a classic American painting, yet more vivid and alive, and still peaceful and reassuring.

This is the view from my room.

I'm thankful for being awakened to it.

☐ Charles Palmisano lived with AIDS for five years before he passed away in September 1991. At the time of his death, he was in his early forties. He had lost contact with his family many years before. Still, he considered the other residents and hospice staff to be members of his extended family. They in turn remember his sense of humor and his "View from My Room," the original of which is framed and displayed in the hospice's living room.

Charles's childhood ambition was to become a writer.

My career is very important to me, and even though I don't tell many people this, I am very proud to be a teacher. I've been a teacher now for 10 years, and where most teachers are bored out of their minds, I now find it the most rewarding thing in my life.

Since I found out I was HIV-positive, I have become a more patient, more loving, more understanding teacher. I listen to my students and take the time to be there for them. I guess I feel that I have very little time to be a good influence on these young students. I really feel now that I can help them not only to be good students but to be good people as well.

Each day makes a difference to me because I know that I am making a difference to them. You don't often get a second chance to be an influence on the future of tomorrow, but I have, and I am taking it to heart.

❑ Eric Steleter was 34 years old when he tested HIV-positive in 1990. His childhood ambition was to be a scientist. At the time of this writing he is still healthy and teaching chemistry to his 10th-grade students, most of whom did not know that he was infected with the virus.

Postal worker Daniel Iszard was diagnosed with AIDS in 1986 at the age of 28. Following his diagnosis, he moved from Alaska to California for treatment. He was initially diagnosed with pneumocystis and tuberculosis. The one constant in his life during his illness was the love and care he received from his younger sister, Jackie.

*D*anny was living and working in Alaska, but he was dating a girl in Los Angeles off and on for about three years. After they broke up, this girl got pregnant, not by Danny, and gave the baby up for adoption. When the baby was three months old, the adoptive parents took it to the doctor because it was always sick. When they discovered the baby had AIDS, they went to Danny's girlfriend and tested her. She was HIV-positive.

Danny had been having trouble with his left eye for a while, and the doctors couldn't figure out what was wrong with him. When Danny's girlfriend told him she was HIV-positive, he went out and got tested. He had *it* big-time and was diagnosed with CMV-retinitis. Needless to say, Danny didn't practice safe sex back then because the thought never entered his mind that he had AIDS. He had guilt about his own girlfriend, and it preyed on his mind a lot.

☐ In 1989, late in the stage of his illness, Danny opted to abruptly stop taking AZT and his other medication. His decline quickly followed.

His girlfriend died, then the baby, then Danny. Three lives are gone because of AIDS.

The only thing, the one deep thing he said to me was, "If I had known that I was going to die so young, I would have done so many other things in my life." We really didn't talk about it much because we would just cry. We all knew what was going on, and we knew what he was going through so we just dealt with it on a daily level.

Our father had passed away. Our mother, I don't have too many good things to say about. We never really knew our mother. I met her when I was 18, and she never saw Danny until six months before he died. He was in the hospital, and she came out here for four days. I feel she did it out of a guilty conscience. At the time I didn't, but now I do. I don't have a lot of respect for her.

Nobody ever came around; his friends never called. His best friend, Rick, called every so often, but not really. They went to see him two days before he passed away. Two of his friends went to the hospice with a six-pack of beer. I wanted to kill them. When they saw him, how incoherent he was, they just got depressed and left.

Danny and I were very, very close. It was hard; it's still hard. I got through it the best I could. I went to work every day. After work I took the bus down there, stayed four or five hours, made dinner, took the bus home, went to bed, and got up and did the same thing, seven days a week.

To a family member of someone with AIDS, I would say, Love them as much as possible. You never know when they're going to be gone. I'm still trying to get over this. I might start sobbing any

26

minute. You just never realize how precious and short life is. I still break down and cry when I hear songs that remind me of Danny.

If you're dealing with someone who has this, you have to deal with what they're going through, deal with what you're going through, and make them as comfortable as possible, which is what I tried to do.

I think everyone should get tested and should practice safe sex. I know that's a lesson I've learned from all of this. I was a drug user, and I've since quit. I got tested, and luckily I'm negative. Still, I will always practice safe sex. Another good thing that came out of this for me is that Danny's home nurse was a gay man who has since become my best friend. He went through all of it with me when nobody else was around. We have a lifetime bond.

Brother, I miss you more than I can say.

—JACKIE ISZARD

Sharon Lund, 42, contracted the AIDS virus in 1984 from her ex-husband, Bill. She would later find out that Bill was bisexual but had never considered himself at risk because his male relationships were only occasional.

When Sharon first discovered that Bill was infected, she called to confront him. He denied that he had tested positive.

I don't think the anger really set in until right before he died in 1990 and he called and admitted the truth. The anger really set in right then and there. I remember thinking, How dare he continue to lie to me for four years while I continued to become progressively ill? For a long time I remained angry. And then I realized that anger was only self-defeating, and I refused to carry it with me any longer. It may seem strange, but having this illness has been the most profound and powerful thing that has ever happened in my life. It has caused me to put my life in order. I've found inner peace. I've found God within me. I've cleared up all my past, all my emotional blockages. Whatever happens from here on out, I'm going to be prepared for it.

Before I got tested, I was a secretary. Today, I'm a spokeswoman for women with HIV. I think it's a crime that the United States government has not looked at the women's issues [pertaining to AIDS]. Women's symptoms are different from men's. We are not getting the care that we need, and our concerns are not being met. When I was diagnosed, the counselor who gave me the news looked at me with tears in his eyes. He said, "I don't know what to tell you. I've never experienced having to tell a woman she's infected." He then proceeded to hand me a handful of pamphlets on AIDS. They were all directed to men.

For the first three years, I was fine. Then, I had severe night sweats, lymphadenopathy, chronic fatigue (which forced me to quit work), wasting syndrome (I lost 23 pounds in six weeks), severe diarrhea, memory loss, herpes, fevers, and candida. Three years ago, when I was extremely ill, they gave me six months to live.

I have only used holistic herbs and vitamins, acupuncture, colonics, visualization, meditation, body dialogue, emotional clearing, a vegetarian diet, and exercise. I think that anything you put in your body, be it aspirin or AZT or anything else, is going to affect another part of your body or another organ. With the toxicity of AZT, there's just no way I would do that to my body. I feel that the herbs and vitamins will build up my immune system, and I won't destroy any of the other organs in my body.

What would I say to other people who are HIV-positive?

The first thing is that they're not alone. That there are other people who are going through it. Not to isolate themselves, and to immediately come out of denial. To find support, whether that support be from family members, from the clergy, from whomever or wherever, find some kind of support. This is not a death sentence. A positive attitude is a part of the healing process. I think the more positive they are, the more uplifted they are, the better their health will be.

29

The main things for me have been meditation and visualization. I think they're what get me through. I always know that God is within me. I still definitely have had some bad days. It was not too many weeks ago that I really wanted to die, I felt so bad. It was just a few days that I went through, but I stayed on my program, and I stayed with my meditation, and it got me through it.

What do I see when I look into the mirror?

Probably the most vibrant and alive and happy person that I've ever seen. For the first time in my life I'm not looking at whether or not my hair is in place or my lipstick is on straight. I am looking at my soul, and I'm pleased with what I see.

—*SHARON LUND*

☐ As of this writing, Sharon was planning to go to Europe to teach people about AIDS. Her childhood ambition was to be a teacher.

With AIDS, she has fulfilled that dream.

I'm 36, but my liver is 90.

I *don't* believe that HIV is the cause of AIDS, so the question of when I was infected with HIV or was diagnosed HIV-positive matters not a whit to me.

I was part of the first HIV testing, and I would assume that I became positive for HIV at the earliest possible opportunity. I lived the classic life-style, which was that I partied hard. And I am famous for being able to rattle off a staggering list of sexually transmitted diseases all in one breath, all of which I had before I was diagnosed with AIDS. I was diagnosed with GRID [Gay-Related Immune Deficiency], which was renamed AIDS a month after I was diagnosed, in the summer of 1982. I was sick with the symptoms that ultimately gave me my official Centers for Disease Control full-blown AIDS diagnosis for at least a year before I was officially diagnosed.

According to the government's own records, there are people who are alive and well who have had AIDS for 12 or 13 years, people retrospectively identified back to 1978 or 1979. I'm sad to say that I don't know any of them personally. For the longest time, I was able to rattle off half a dozen names of people who were my elders, the AIDS class of 1981. I'm from the class of 1982. Unfortunately, they have all, at least the ones I knew, died. I am now the longest living survivor I know.

I have a lot of friends who are New Age [oriented] and who are holistic. They just don't know what to make of me. I eat like a pig and I eat really well. But sugar is one of my three or four main reasons for living. I'm a classic Coca-Cola addict. Aside from yoga, I have not dabbled much in so-called alternative, homeopathic forms of medicine. Many long-term survivors of AIDS have. I am simply not among them.

I am pleased to say that I have never taken a single AZT pill. I'm very Western science-oriented, even though I disagree with AZT. I do take about 52 pills a day. My strategy for the last several years has been prophylactic. There are about half a dozen opportunistic infections that account for about 95 percent of all AIDS deaths. With the exceptions of the cancers, specifically KS, five of the six diseases [any one of which constitute an official AIDS diagnosis by the CDC] are exquisitely ripe for prophylactic treatment strategies in exactly the same way that we've discovered you can pretty effectively prevent pneumocystis. I take pills to prevent decimated herpes, CMV [cytomegalovirus], and herpes simplex one and two. I take antifungal medications to prevent cryptococcal meningitis. I take anti-TB drugs to prevent MAC [mycobacterium avium complex]. And, of course, I take Bactrim to prevent PCP. I feel very strongly that if more people with AIDS would approach their treatment strategy from a prophylactic standpoint, we would see dramatic increases in the number of survivors. It's not that I'm not concerned with the underlying immune deficiency itself. I just have not seen any evidence that any of the currently available drugs, or drugs from the underground or holistic world, have any kind of reliable and beneficial effects on increasing your T-cells.

My doctor put me on Bactrim in 1982, and I felt dramatically, immediately better. No one has suggested that Bactrim is a cure for cryptosporidium, my diagnosing illness, but my improvement was dramatic. I also have KS, which I've had for at least three years. And my main problem is bacterial pneumonia, which I get religiously every September. If I could afford it, I would have gamma-globulin shots, but I can't, so I don't. My last bout with bacterial pneumonia lasted five months. I had a hell of a time getting rid of it, but I finally did.

Before I was diagnosed, I was a slut and proud of it. If I had had my wits about me I would have tried to make some money from it. I was giving it away for free. I was a very active credit to the sexual revolution. And I'm not really joking. I worked as a legal secretary. But almost all the rest of the time was spent in the pursuit of sex. I didn't have many friends. I didn't belong to any organizations. I worked. I slept. I had sex. I went to school at Boston University, and I told everybody, including myself, that I moved to New York to pursue my singing career. But in fact, I didn't sing very much, and instead, I pursued my career as a slut. And I was very, very good at that career.

I am completely different now than I was. "Major life-style change" does not quite capture the magnitude. I know it sounds silly and simple, but most people with AIDS, and others with some state of immunodeficiency, follow their grandmother's advice, including me. Eat right, get plenty of sleep, fall in love, and avoid sexually transmitted diseases. Unfortunately, because the federal research effort has been such a monumental failure, there isn't much better advice than that. I happen to feel that's pretty good advice.

I know more long-term AIDS survivors than anyone else in the world—for the sad but simple reason that I'm probably the only one who's gone in search of them—and I noticed among long-term survivors that *all of them were not yet done with life*. All of them had at least one major project that they wanted to complete before they died. I restudied the literature of extraordinary cancer survivors and found that *a reason to live* is one of the defining characteristics of survivors of cancer.

It has been incredibly frustrating to me to see people lose respect for the distinction between being sick and not being sick. When you have HIV, you are not necessarily sick, nor will you necessarily get sick.

I'm not denying that there are similarities between the experience of finding out you're HIV-positive and finding out that you have AIDS. Given what the world believes about HIV, people who find out that they're HIV-positive do, in fact, suffer many of the same emotional experiences that people who have full-blown AIDS experience and are subject to pretty much the same discrimination. I'm merely begging people to honor the distinction between having HIV and feeling well, and having AIDS and not feeling very well. To me, to use the terms interchangeably is deeply offensive. And I also believe that, in a sense, it can become a self-fulfilling prophecy, you know? The HIV-equals-AIDS conveyor-belt theory encourages people to take toxic drugs at an early point, which, in my opinion, tends to bring on the symptoms of AIDS sooner than if one did nothing. I believe that AZT speeds up the process of T-cell depletion.

The first thing I would tell a person who's HIV-positive is to at least consider the possibility that they will never get sick, that they will grow old and grumpy and live to collect social security.

A person who has an AIDS diagnosis is quite clearly much, much sicker, and there's no getting around the fact that once you've had an AIDS-defining opportunistic infection, your statistical probability of dying sooner, rather than later, is undeniable. But my whole message for the past two years has been that nothing in your lab report can tell you whether you're going to survive or not.

Since no one knows for certain what their fate is, post-AIDS, it makes rational sense to live as if you were going to be among the survivors. If you live as if you're doomed, it saps your will to fight, and you might bring it on sooner. The quality of whatever time you have left on earth will probably be worse than it would be if you could somehow muster some optimism.

What would I say to other people with AIDS?

Fight the fatalism that is so inextricably built into the way we think and talk about AIDS. And one way of fighting that fatalism, and a sort of general piece of advice, is to doubt all things, including anything I say in this interview. Take nothing at face value. Each one of us is biochemically, philosophically unique. What may work for one person may not work for another.

To each person who is ill, I say, ultimately, *you* must take responsibility for the choices that you make. It's you who will experience the side effects. It's your life that will be shortened or lengthened. But the problem with my recommendation is that it is kind of contrary to human nature. Especially when you're ill, you have the tendency to reach out and rely on the goodwill of others, to assume that they have your best interests at heart. Unfortunately, the track record on AIDS will demonstrate pretty much the opposite. And so when a person is at their weakest or their lowest is precisely the time when they need to keep their wits about them, because they will be making life-or-death treatment choices. They need to do their homework.

What that has meant for me is seeking out—and it's very painful to do this—people who have diverse opinions, often people who passionately believe the opposite of what I believe. I go to them and I say, "Tell me again why you have looked at the same evidence

I have looked at and have come to the opposite conclusion." I really want to understand the different viewpoints that surround AIDS. Most people prefer to decide what they believe, seek out other people who believe that way, and then convince themselves that everyone thinks that way. It's very threatening to most people to actually aggressively seek out people who disagree with them. But I would argue that with AIDS, the stakes are so high you need to test your beliefs. It's hard work, but it's worth it.

What do I still want to accomplish?

I wouldn't mind getting involved in other political struggles, specifically, the feminist struggle. I really feel that I owe women, in particular the women's health-care movement, a huge debt for what they taught me at the crucial early beginnings of my own struggle to negotiate with the health-care systems. I mean, my idea of a good time is to sit on the toilet and read obscure French feminist theory. I just can't get enough of it. I love, love feminism, and so you can say that my goal is to live long enough to see the feminist revolution won, which will be a very long time, indeed.

There are things that I would like to accomplish but that I'm not necessarily going after or think will be likely. I'm poor white trash. I come from a lower-middle-class Midwestern background. In the last 10 years I've met some really wealthy people and people who are financially secure, who don't know what it's like to wonder where their next month's rent would come from. I would love, before I die, to know that kind of financial security. I'm not doing anything at all to bring that about. I mean, it's not like you can make a living as an openly gay artist. I live on disability now.

I have fantasies. I love, love, love to cook. Actually, I love to bake more than cook, although I love to cook, also. And I often get lost in the reverie of not so much opening a restaurant but of opening a really nice bakery. Or just a sort of coffeehouse where people would be encouraged to just sit all day and read and hang out. Maybe there would be poetry readings and lectures, and really, really good food . . .

And maybe a song or two from me at the piano.

—MICHAEL CALLEN

☐ Michael Callen is a long-term survivor of AIDS, controversial AIDS activist, singer, songwriter, and author. His book, the succinctly titled *Surviving AIDS,* was published by HarperCollins in 1990.

When asked what his childhood ambition was, Michael responded, "Like every third homosexual, I wanted to be Barbra Streisand. My fantasy was that after I left my podunk town and moved to the big city, I was gonna go to some obscure cabaret, find a '20s or '30s torch song, slow it way down, and instantly be signed by Columbia Records."

Since his diagnosis Michael has recorded two albums and as of this writing is working on another.

My name is Todd Husted. Three years ago I was working at AIDS Project Los Angeles as a phone buddy for patients diagnosed with the AIDS virus. One of my calls one day was to Craig Royce. I explained to him what the program was, and with his permission, I told him I would be calling him every other week to check up on him and see how he was doing. He said that would be fine. After I hung up, I wasn't sure how he really felt, because he had sounded so curt and distant, but I knew this was to be expected, given the circumstances. I called the following week. He was surprised to hear from me, but his attitude was much more relaxed and open.

A strange thing happened in the weeks that followed as Craig and I continued to converse over the phone. For the first time in my life I began to experience a sense of freedom that I had never felt before; an ability to discuss openly, and without fear of being judged, my innermost feelings about myself, my life, and my "life-style." With no apologies and no regrets.

Craig said he felt the same way. We talked about everything. But what each of us knew and would not admit was that this newfound freedom was the result of never having met face-to-face. The phone had liberated us. It had given each of us a sense of protective anonymity that we might not have otherwise achieved. But what was wrong with that? I asked myself. And the answer came back loud and clear: Nothing!

I wanted to meet Craig. This was something the program encouraged us strongly *not* to do. Be caring, be supportive, but don't get too involved. Guess what? It was too late. I felt that if I didn't meet Craig I would regret it for the rest of my life.

I told Craig I wanted to meet him. He was apprehensive. No surprise there. Neither one of us wanted to risk destroying what we had created. What if we didn't like each other? What if we were turned off by each other's looks? So many what-ifs. I told Craig I had made a list of what I was looking for in a relationship. The list was two pages long. Craig laughed and said he could never come up with two pages of anything, let alone a list of the ideal relationship. But he finally went the distance. When we started exchanging the items on our laundry lists, we were both amazed to find how similar they were. It was as if each of us had been looking over the other's shoulder as we put pen to paper. The only thing different was the order of our priorities. But after all, lists can be rearranged.

Craig said he would send me a photograph. I panicked. I thought, My God, I don't have a picture to send him! What I was really saying to myself was, I didn't have a flattering picture. Every insecurity I had came rushing to the surface. What if he didn't like the beard? He would think, of course, "No chin." Well, at least I hadn't told him I was a buffed and beautiful bodybuilder. At least I had had the good sense not to tell him much of anything about how I looked.

Two days later Craig's picture arrived. It was love at first sight. And then we met. The first thing Craig said was that he already knew what I looked like, he didn't need a picture. And the beard was just fine with him, chin or no chin. We were both very nervous.

I showed him around my apartment and babbled nonstop about where I had gotten this chair, and where I had gotten that mirror, and who had given me the dining-room table, and so on. I was sure Craig wasn't going to remember a thing I was saying.

Craig had plans for us to go to a street fair, but as we continued to talk and work through our fear of what was happening, or what might happen, the day just disappeared on us. We did manage to go to one of Craig's favorite restaurants for dinner. That night I knew I wanted to share the rest of my life with Craig, to have him share with me what was left of his life.

Eventually, Craig moved in. No sooner had that happened than we realized we needed a bigger place. We found the perfect apartment. And then Craig got sick. Very sick. How can you even begin to deal with the horror of AIDS when you can't even pronounce half of the multiple and torturous medical words used to describe this gruesome disease? Pneumocystis carinii pneumonia, toxoplasmosis, cytomegaloviris-retinitis, oral candidiasis. It's bad enough with the terms that you do understand, or think you understand, like AIDS dementia, pancreatitis, seizures, rectal hemorrhaging. On one occasion Craig was bleeding rectally, the blood literally pouring out of his rectum. I thought to myself, My God, he's going to bleed to death before the paramedics get here! *If* they ever get here.

And the medication. There were times when Craig was taking as many as 20 different pills a day. We had to write down each individual pill and when they were taken just to keep track of them all. It became a full-time job monitoring the callous, lackadaisical doctors and getting the insurance company to fulfill its contractual obligations, a never-ending nightmare-blizzard of paperwork.

My anger has grown at a government that has dragged its feet on funding for AIDS research, realizing that by the time it will touch the lives of those people who need it the most, it will be too late. How can I, a lay person, possibly keep up on the latest in drug research? And why did the doctor fail to mention that one of the side effects of DDI could result in seizures? And it did.

Through the grapevine we heard about passive immunotherapy. We made an appointment to see the only doctor who was practicing this experimental procedure. When we walked into his office and saw how lavishly it was decorated and beheld how well-dressed the doctor was, we should have known where our fee of $2,250 was going. His attitude was, "Don't worry about the bill. The insurance company will take care of it." You couldn't get in the door if you weren't able to come up with the full amount—and of course, in the end, the treatment was a total failure.

But the one thing that cannot be taken away from me by all of this is my memories.

I remember the time we met Ed, one of our best friends, for dinner. I went in first to see if Ed had arrived. I left Craig outside the restaurant because he was feeling extremely weak that night and he wanted a few extra minutes to get his strength back. Ed came out of the restaurant with me to help Craig inside. When Craig saw Ed, he lifted his arms to wave a greeting, and just as he did, his pants fell to the ground. We laughed about that one all through dinner.

We shared wonderful trips to Carmel, San Francisco, and Kauai. Together, we worked through some of the hardest things we would ever have to deal with, all the while growing closer and deepening our love for each other. Who would have thought that at 31 years of age we would be confronted with the bizarre-sounding legalese of "durable power of attorney" for medical care, drafting a will, and the ultimate finality of planning a funeral? But then this was also

41

softened by the fact that Craig's beautiful parents accepted me from day one as their own.

I can remember getting notes on the bathroom mirror from Craig saying, "What would I be without you? Who would I be without you? Would I dare be without you? Love, Little Schnook."

Today Craig's life has been reduced to the minimal denominator. We have breakfast together, and then he goes back to bed. He spends the day with his companion, Mason. He's become increasingly disoriented and forgetful, so he needs someone with him all the time. Craig had a lot of friends and business associates before he became ill. But as the AIDS virus ravaged him, as his physical and mental condition became more pronounced, the less frequent their visits became. The people he loved the most, at a time when he needed them the most, just disappeared.

I come home after work and make dinner. Then Craig goes back to bed and is usually asleep by nine o'clock. Through all of this I have been forced to grow up much faster than I ever wanted to. I've stopped playing the games I used to play, the emotional mind games that we all play. Life is too short. And you realize just how fast it can be taken away. Tell people you love them while there's still time. Because 30 minutes of something wonderful is better than a lifetime of nothing special.

Thank you, Craig, for giving me those 30 wonderful minutes.

□ On July 11, 1991, after he so eloquently expressed the words above, Todd Husted lost Craig to AIDS.
A few months later, Todd, who is HIV-negative, was interviewed again for this project. Today, he still works as an AIDS volunteer.

I went into it with my eyes open. People said, "Don't go into it, you're setting yourself up to be hurt." I thought, "Why not take the risk? You're going to get hurt anyway in life." I thought I would enjoy it for as long as I could.

What would I say to other AIDS caregivers?

Set boundaries. Take care of yourself. Tell people what you need. Toward the end, it got to the point where I called a friend and said, "Look, this is what's happening; can I rely on you or not?" In the end, you need to know who is going to be there and who is not. That's all part of taking care of yourself. Actually, most people said, "No problem." A lot of people said if I needed to take time off, to just call them. I called them on it. I was very honest and I said, "Look, this is what I want, this is what I need."

You also have to communicate with the doctor. Make sure you have doctors you can trust, whom you can ask questions without their getting defensive.

It took me about six months to get the durable power of attorney for medical care. The things that are most important are things like wills, durable power of attorney for medical care, funeral arrangements. I made Craig feel very guilty because he didn't want to talk about it, and I said, "It's very selfish of you to die and not let me know what you want." Talk about it and do it and get it over with.

And you're never ready for them to die. No matter how prepared you are, you're never ready. We had done everything. We talked about it. But you're never ready for the inevitable.

The thing that has helped me has been the support group that Jackie Black runs through Northern Lights. It's absolutely incredible. Jackie feels that the major bereavement should take 8 to 10 weeks. You do exercises, you make a list, you make amends. It's somewhat like a 12-step program. But it's very confrontive, and it has definitely been the thing that has gotten me through. I would definitely suggest a support group. The first month and a half, you're just numb. I constantly picked up the phone to call Craig.

The reality for me didn't start hitting until about two months after his death.

My life is just now starting to come back into, I guess, well, *living.*

—*TODD HUSTED*

On October 1, 1991, actor Dack Rambo, 49, gave Hollywood a jolt by announcing that he was HIV-positive and was quitting his job on the daytime television drama "Another World." The former costar of "Dallas" further announced his intention to devote his time and efforts to publicly speaking out and fighting the disease.

He expands on that pledge and pursues that commitment with the following words.

Going public with my diagnosis was the most frightening decision I had ever faced. After the initial shock, I knew what I wanted to do and what I had to do. I decided to leave New York and my television family to come home [to Los Angeles] and devote my life to the battle against AIDS and HIV in any way I could.

I know my ability to step forward and be public about my diagnosis was made easier by the love and support that I knew would embrace me.

Despite the false security of days gone by, this has never been exclusively a disease of the so-called high-risk groups. HIV is a disease of the human race, and finally, thank God, it is being acknowledged as such.

I salute Magic Johnson for erasing some of the stigma that people with HIV face, but I also say thank you and salute so many others for starting a battle cry and continuing the war against ignorance and illness. Together in our industry we are uniquely able to raise funds and raise consciousness.

—DACK RAMBO

The feeling that I had when I was told that I had AIDS was one of great disappointment—for me and for my lover, David.

Initially, I thought that I only had a few months to live, five at the most. It's now been over four years. After my diagnosis, I decided that I didn't want to be a walking, talking person with AIDS, so I went back to work. I worked as a manager at the Amtrak ticket office. I tried to lead as normal a life as I could.

In March of 1990, I stopped working. I have had pneumocystis four times, CMV in my lungs, and CMV-retinitis. But I've been very optimistic. I have always been an optimistic person, and I also have a very deep Christian faith. I've never been bitter. I've never said, Why me? My feelings have always been, Why *not* me?

I've had very few days when I was really depressed. I just take it in stride and do the best I can. I hope for the best. It's actually been a remarkable experience for me because I've seen so much love and caring, and so many people have been good to me. I've never had an uncomfortable or bad reaction from anyone. My family has been wonderful and so has my lover.

I've just learned a lot about appreciating life. It's been quite an education. It has also brought me closer to my parents. I always look for the blessings and the rewards of the illness. I know that everyone doesn't feel that way—a lot of people have had people turn on them. But I've always been kind to people, and I just feel like I'm being rewarded for that now with all the kindness and love I'm getting. Some of the blessings I feel that I've gotten since I became ill are the great doctors and nurses who have cared for me and the new friends I now have that I met through AIDS Project Los Angeles and other AIDS-related support groups.

I am now able to hear a concert or see a fireworks display and appreciate the beauty. At times, I weep at some of these beautiful blessings. I know that this may sound odd, but I would never have wanted to miss all of that.

I'll never say, I wish this never happened.

—MARK GIFFORD

☐ Mark Gifford died on March 9, 1992. His childhood ambition had been to be a comedian. It was a goal that he, in some ways, fulfilled. "I've put my sense of humor to better use," Mark said shortly before his death. "It's gotten me through a lot of hard times."

Mark Gifford was 34 years old. His friends will never forget his spirit or his smile.

$\mathcal{N}$ow I know what it's like to be in a prison camp. It's not the disease; it's the way people have responded to it. I feel ostracized.

Before I got sick, superficial things were really important to me. I wanted to have the best clothes. I wanted to have the best body. I wanted to have the best tan. I wanted to have the nicest car and the most money. I wanted to be popular, and I was. After I found out I had AIDS, I was rejected by the gay community in West Hollywood. Suddenly they had no time for me, these people whom I thought were my friends. One day this guy came up to me at the gym and said, "You know, Chris, you'd better not spread this disease"—as if I needed to be told that! That really hurt me. The attitude is, I don't have it yet, so I'm going to stay away from you. I thought that I would've been welcomed with open arms. Since that day I have not gone back to the gym.

My work was also very important to me. If I had to work 14 hours a day, that was OK with me. I didn't want to be a failure. I wanted to make my parents and my lover, Neal, proud of me.

Looking back on it now, it was all meaningless.

I just had brain surgery. They inserted a shunt into my brain. The doctors told me that I would have a stroke if I didn't have the operation, so I had it. The operation wasn't too bad, but the rest of it was awful. There I was, hooked up to all these machines, and I felt like some kind of a monster. In intensive care, there were mix-ups in my medication, they had to put a catheter in me every two hours, and I was having all this pain. I didn't know what was going on. I thought I was going to die.

I met my friend Mark Gifford at a support group for people with CMV-retinitis. I'm blind in one eye. We became instant friends. Mark made me feel like, Hey, it's not so bad having AIDS. He had been through *everything* there is with AIDS, and I watched him deteriorate month after month, day after day. And I thought, selfishly, "God, don't let what's happening to Mark happen to me." But Mark was more worried about me than he was about himself. I spoke with him the night before I went into the hospital to have the brain operation. He had a fever of 104 degrees, but all he could talk about was me, and the surgery I was about to have.

I was in the hospital after the surgery when I learned that Mark had checked into the same hospital in a room close to mine. I went to visit him, but he was already out of it. He was dying. I was in his room five minutes after he passed away, and I knew that he was already gone. Lying on the bed was just his shell. I don't know if there is a heaven, hell, or whatever. I feel like I'm in purgatory, doing my time. Mark, though, went straight to heaven. I know that he did.

Mark was not the type of person I would've been friends with before I got sick. He was tall, lanky, and not great looking. He wore polyester pants, for God's sake! But I learned that these were superficial things. One day Mark said to me, "Chris, you would never have been my friend if I wasn't sick." I said, "You're probably right." And you know what? I think Mark was one of the best friends I ever had.

50

Now I worry all the time, Oh, God! What if Neal gets sick?

For years I had put off getting the HIV test, and when I found out I was positive, it was in the worst possible way. I was rushed to the hospital emergency room and was later diagnosed with meningitis and encephalitis. The following week I was told that I had CMV-retinitis and AIDS. I should've gotten tested sooner. My father is a doctor, and I should've been more aware of what was going on in my body. But you know what? I truly thought that I was past the point where I had to worry. I had been in a long-term relationship with Neal, and I thought I was in the clear. I thought we were both safe. I learned that *nobody* is safe.

I've become more realistic. I also think I've become a better person. I don't live in this fairy-tale world anymore. AIDS is real. Meningitis is real. Not being able to walk without assistance is real. I used to love to gossip about other people. Now I have no time for that. I'm too busy trying to live. Sometimes I feel like people are just waiting for me to die. But I feel like a gladiator. I'm not ready to go down.

What would I say to others?

Believe me, I've tried everything, done everything, and one of the things I've learned is that the healing has to start from within. *Forgive* yourself. With AIDS, there shouldn't be blame. Let go of it.

I also feel it's important to have a schedule. I'm involved in an experimental project called Partners in which 20 elderly people are paired with 20 people with AIDS. The hope is that we'll all learn from one another. Every day, even if I don't feel like it, I go there. I know that it's good for me. They call me the mayor there because I'm always organizing things. I always lead the exercise class. We work out while sitting in chairs. I wonder what the guys back at the gym would say?

One more thing: Each day, give yourself a little project to do.

Even if it's just taking a shower or shaving or getting a haircut or making a meat loaf. One day I went out and got my ear pierced. Ever since I was a little boy I had wanted to get my ear pierced. That might seem silly to some people, but to me it was a dream fulfilled.

What do I see when I look into the mirror?

Two years ago I saw a handsome young man with a great body who also happened to be sometimes a nasty and spoiled brat. Today I look into the mirror and I see a nice person who has paid his debt to society. I see a person who has always been nice but who didn't know how to be. I wish that it didn't take getting sick to find that person, but it did. As for my looks, I look into the mirror and I say to myself, You know what? You look damned good!

—CHRISTOPHER ESPOSITO

☐ Christopher Esposito was 31 years old when he was diagnosed with AIDS in August 1990. He lost the sight in his right eye and as of this writing he has difficulty walking and maintaining his balance. Still, Chris is a gourmet cook, and he looks forward to the day when he can entertain his friends with a meal of stuffed shells and sweet Italian sausages.

Chris's childhood ambition was to be a musical star on Broadway. His present ambition, in his own words, is "to have a good day."

(Editor's note: Christopher Esposito is the author's companion and significant other. Neal and Chris have been together for nine years.)

The reason I went in to be tested was because my lover, Tim, had tested HIV-positive and his life began to fall apart. My life changed to taking care of him.

We had been living in Fort Wayne, Indiana, a negative sort of environment, so he had to remain in the closet. I don't even think he told his doctor he was gay. He had had shingles in 1986, and the doctor just told him, "Oh, this happens occasionally. I wouldn't worry about it." Of course, now we know better. Anyway, as he moved up the career ladder, he started developing ulcers, which the doctor couldn't understand because none of the treatments were working. It turned out later that CMV was beginning to eat away his stomach.

Well, we moved to Chicago and lived there for three years. In Chicago, Tim finally gave in and went to get tested. He was going to be 33 when he died. I was 27. I had been with him for seven and a half years. Before that I had had a couple of two- or three-month relationships. I had been around. But this was definitely my longest relationship. I mean, I have his initials tattooed on my arms, you know?

When you have your chosen partner die in your arms, it really clears out a lot of bullshit. You know, all your life you're told it's important that you get a job, that you make lots of money, that you own lots of property, and that you have children. When you face the death of someone you've chosen to love, you learn what really is important. If someone offered me a million-dollar recording contract tomorrow, yeah, I'd do it, but at the same time, I have the satisfaction of knowing that I'm loved and that the world exists, and that there *are* reasons for things.

My biggest fear used to be, before I came out, that my family would reject me. And you know what? My family has been amazing. My coming out changed their perception about how many grandchildren they were gonna have, but other than that, they've been very supporting. It's been amazing to me that they love me this much, that they've done this much. When Tim died, they flew in from all over the country within 12 hours to be there for me—from Tallahassee, from Indianapolis, and from Santa Barbara.

What would I say to other people?

I don't care who you are, if you haven't been tested, get tested. Continue to be tested. Knowledge is the only way to fight this thing. Second of all, take command of your own health care. Don't sit back and let a doctor tell you, "Well, you've got HIV, you're gonna die." I don't think that any real doctor would say that these days. But when we were in Fort Wayne, it was a very real fear for Tim. The doctors didn't know much about this disease, and they still don't. Everybody's guessing. But at least they've done some things that are able to stave it off for awhile. It's important to educate yourself about what's out there. And if you don't like your doctor, you don't think that he's giving you the right answers, then go to another one.

As for safe sex, it's the only kind of sex to have these days. No orgasm is worth dying for. You know, I think that anybody who is continuing to have unprotected sex should be forced to walk through an AIDS ward. They should watch these people spit up bile with their last breath, watch these people not be able to control themselves, watch these people shake, and watch these people babble on to people who aren't even existing on the earth anymore. And then tell me that an orgasm is worth it.

What was my childhood ambition?

David Bowie's *Young Americans* album got me through the wild teenage years, where your whole mind is rushing. I always wanted to be able to write a song that would mean something, that would help someone get through a tough night or a tough time. That's what I wanted. I wanted to be a big rock star. I wouldn't mind all the cars and stuff, you know? But the main reason I wanted to get into music was to help other people. I know that music helped me get through some tough times. I'd like to teach the world to sing— and better.

—BRIAN BALDUS

☐ Brian Baldus, 29, was diagnosed with cyptococcal meningitis and AIDS during Labor Day weekend of 1991.

Weeks after he received his diagnosis, Brian's nephew was born. Says Brian, "You know, I've seen so much death. Little Jack Spurtz being born was quite important to me. I have a sense of hope for the future a little bit. It recharged my batteries."

Brian is currently rehearsing and performing with his rock-and-roll band named Love Life.

For a year and a half, while his friends were outside playing ball, eight-year-old Troy Blocker was fighting for his life.

I was seven months pregnant when Troy was born at Cedars-Sinai Hospital in Los Angeles in 1981. He had to get a blood transfusion. Then they said on the news in 1987 that if your child had been born at Cedars-Sinai between 1980 and 1985, something like that, and had received blood, there was a possibility of contamination with the AIDS virus. They had a number on the screen and said, "Call this number to have your child tested." I called the next day.

Over the years, Troy had had pneumonia, asthma, and ear infections, but nobody ever thought that this could be AIDS. I mean, he never looked very sick. He was always very plump, on the chubby side.

In January of 1988 they told me he was HIV-positive.

When I first found out, my first reaction was, Oh, my God! This is a dream! This isn't real! and, Should I tell him?

The first thing that goes on in your mind is, is he going to die? Then, when we were going back to the doctor for a second test, I thought, well, we're going to have to be coming here a lot, and he's going to need to know why. We were in the car—me, Troy, and his younger brother, Aaron—and I went, "Well, you guys, what do you know about AIDS? What do you think AIDS is?" And they said, "Well, it's a disease and people get sick and you could die from it."

I waited a little longer until I brought it up again. Finally, I took Troy into the bathroom, and we were sitting there talking when I said, "Troy, remember when we talked about AIDS? What would you do if you knew somebody who had it?" And he said, "Well, I don't know. I don't know if I'd play with them anymore." Then we talked about how you can get it, and I said, "Well, there's somebody we know who has it." He said, "Who?" And I said, "You."

I told him how he had gotten it, and he wanted to know who knew about it. Then he said, "Well, I don't want to tell my friends. I don't want them to know. Because if they know they'll tease me and say things like, 'Troy has AIDS.' And I don't want them to do that."

And then I told him, "I love you very much, and any time you need to talk about it, we can talk about it." Later on he came to me and said, "Do I *really* have it?" And I said, "Yeah." Then he asked, "Am I going to die?" And I said, "Well, some people live a long time with it. And some people die." I just kind of left it like that.

I was a single parent at the time. I had separated from my first husband, Troy's father. When I first found out there was a remote possibility that Troy might be infected, I called his father up. I had never called him, but I figured that this was his son and he needed to know. I didn't get much of a response.

I had just gotten a promotion at my job and they were really strict, so the doctors had to write a letter telling them what was going on with Troy. Their basic response was, "Well, OK, we're really sorry. However, this is your job." It was real hard for me to get the time to take Troy to his doctor's appointments. My job would go, "Isn't there somebody else that can take him? Do *you* have to take him?" On the one hand I felt like, well, I needed the job to keep the medical insurance. On the other hand, I was torn because I felt I wasn't taking care of business with my son.

One day I was looking at Troy in his underwear while he was getting ready to take a bath. I said to myself, God, he's getting really skinny. His weight just started dropping off. The doctor told me that he was starving to death, even if he was eating. He was also getting real tired and would have night sweats.

By this time I had met a man, Aideen, who told me, "I'll be there with you all the way"—and he was. He was a godsend. Where did he come from? Because I'm not this raving beauty, you know? Anyway, I was feeling really angry, because while I was at work, this wonderful man was taking care of and doing all these wonderful things for my son. I thought, but *I'm* Troy's mother, *I'm* the one who should be here. Why am I letting a job dictate to me about being with my son? And I figured if it was their kid, they'd be right there. So, I just called up a friend who was a supervisor at my job and said, "Look, I don't care anymore. I'm not coming back. If they want to fire me, fine."

After Troy would go to bed, I would look at all his baby pictures. I would watch him while he slept and I'd kiss him. Just the thought that he wouldn't be there . . .

In January he went into the hospital to have a catheter surgically put in his chest. Right after he got out of the hospital, we could see that he was giving up. He didn't want to eat and would just lay there wasting away. We sat down and told him, "Troy, if you don't fight this, you're gonna die real fast." And he kind of snapped out of it.

But later, after we came back from a trip to Louisiana, it was like, He's not going to be around much longer. One time we were at the hospital and I said to him, "Troy, if you just get tired and you don't feel like fighting anymore, it's OK." He looked at me and said, "But I don't want to die." Later on that night, I said to him, "Are you afraid to die?" He said, "Yeah." I told him, "You know, Troy, it's really not that bad."

One of the things that Troy and his brother, Aaron, and I used to do was to sit around and go, "We wish we had a house," because we lived in an apartment. It was like, "God, if we had a house it would be so cool," you know? "Everybody can have their own room and we'd have this backyard, and we'd have a pet." There were times when we didn't have any money and I would go, "Boys, we just don't have any money. What can we do?" And so we'd go on walks or pack a lunch and go spend all day at the beach. Or just sit and talk and fantasize about one day getting a house. In the Bible it says, "In my father's house there are many mansions"—and I thought about that. I told Troy that night in the hospital, "Troy, it's going to be so cool. You're gonna have your own house. You can have everything in it that you want, and all the food you want to eat." I just laid it on. When I put him to bed, he said, "Mommy, you made me so happy." "Why?" I said. And he said, "You told me I'm going to have my own house. I'm not afraid to die anymore."

At the end, Troy was having problems controlling his bowels. One night he came into our room and said, "Can I get into bed with you and Daddy?" because by then both of the kids were calling Aideen "Daddy." After we all dozed off, Aideen said to me, "Shevawn, I need you to help me. Troy messed up the bed." Aideen put him in the shower, washed him all off, got him dressed in his pajamas, and put him back to bed.

It was around four in the morning. I walked into the room to tell Troy that it was OK, that we weren't angry at him. He was facing the wall. "Troy, it's OK," I said. "Troy?" But he was just making these noises. I called to Aideen, "Something's not right." Aideen turned him over and Troy had this really strange look on his face, staring off. Even if you lined up your eyes with his, he didn't see you, and every time he heard my voice, the noises would just get louder and louder.

I jumped on the phone and called the doctor. She said, "Shevawn, this is *it.*" I dropped the phone and I ran back to his side, going, "Troy, Mommy's here. We love you. We love you!" Aideen was going, "Hold on, hold on." His breathing was getting kind of heavy, kind of quick. I don't know how long we spent there, telling him, "We love you, we love you." Aideen kept listening to his chest. And finally, I just said, "Troy, look for the house. Look for the house." Just like that, his eyes kind of looked up. And then he died.

The first year after Troy's death was sheer hell for Aaron. He just didn't know what to do with himself. He didn't want to go into the room he had shared with Troy, even though we painted it and changed things around. He didn't go outside a lot. He was lost. His brother was gone. I felt so bad because I didn't know how to help him. When Troy died, Aaron said, "I thought we'd grow up together."

Now Aaron, who's eight, will tell you about AIDS in a minute. He's gotten a lot wiser about it. He thinks nothing about telling you that he had a brother named Troy who died of AIDS. And if he hears you say something stupid about it, he's going to tell you about it. He's not going to let you get away with it. He really doesn't let you get away with any crap.

As for me, I still have these dreams. They're so real. There's this one when Troy comes in to tell me that he's OK. He looks really healthy and he says, "Well, I have to go." I say, "I want to go with you," and then this woman steps in and says, "You can't go now." I definitely think there's something . . . I definitely think there's something else going on, you know?

—*SHEVAWN AVILA*

☐ Troy Blocker died on June 16, 1989. Today his mother, Shevawn Avila, is an AIDS volunteer with Tuesday's Child, a service organization for children with HIV and their families.

She is also married to Aideen, and as of this writing they were anticipating the birth of their first child.

I consider being HIV-positive a series of highs and lows, lessons to be learned. I look at it as, What can I get out of this experience? Just when I think I have things figured out, I want to prepare myself for a new lesson that might come along. I don't want to get too spiritual on you, and I won't. But that's the way it is.

Life is a learning experience, and I think it's good to find yourself developing a new interest. I became a voracious reader right when I found out I was positive, and I can't really understand why.

Find those interests and really cultivate them. I think if you do develop them, you're really listening to an inner voice. Sooner or later, all these new pieces of the puzzle in your life will be put together when you need them. I have happily discovered that is the case with me.

I'm a waiter, but I invested some money in stocks and I started studying the stock market. I found great satisfaction in that and also in dancing, reading, and crossword puzzles. I think you need to go with these feelings and go with your inner self. And, God knows, if you have an emotional or physical uprising, which I did last week, then you'll really be able to heal yourself from within.

—*ANSON FARRAR*

☐ Anson Farrar, 33, tested HIV-positive in July 1988 after losing a lot of weight. He has been on AZT for two years, sees an acupuncturist, takes herbs, and has changed his diet. His childhood ambition was to become an actor, a goal he shelved in favor of "other forms of creative expression" after receiving his diagnosis. One such form is a monthly newsletter which he circulates to family and friends to share, in his words, "the good, bad, courage, fear, pain, growth, change, and lessons learned" in his battle with HIV. The following is a portion of a letter Anson wrote to his parents. It is reprinted below with his permission.

"I often want to rise early, go out and get a paper, check my stock, and do the crossword over a croissant and a cup of tea. These are interests developed after I tested positive. How exciting! How surprising! Knowledge is empowerment, and interests are essential!"

The Reverend John Heschle of the Church of St. Anne in
Morrison, Illinois, is an AIDS buddy. His buddy, Ed, was
diagnosed with HIV in 1987. Ed was stricken with
pneumocystis, Kaposi's sarcoma, CMV-retinitis,
tuberculosis, and bronchitis.

*E*d lived with his mother and father in the Chicago area. It was
very difficult for them. They were very, very fearful. They tried and
tried to be educated, but they also slipped back and feared things
about the disease that they didn't know or weren't being told. As
buddies, Ed and I appeared together in an interview for a Rockford,
Illinois, television show. They colored out his face, but they interviewed me as who I was. There was a little bit of upset in his family
because of the show. There *is* fear in the rural areas.

Ed would say that he was a bisexual who wanted to be heterosexual. I would say he was a homosexual who had been greatly shamed into believing that the only thing acceptable, the only way to get to a higher power, to God, was through a heterosexual lifestyle. He had two ex-wives and three children. He also married a man in San Francisco. Obviously, there were great struggles in his life over this issue.

Because he had been in and out of the gay "life-style," Ed encouraged his parents to think that he could change his sexuality. His first sexual experiences were with men in college. Later he went on to discover that he could also have an enjoyable sex life with women. Then, when he went back to being gay, his parents were unable to accept it.

Ed was a very good father. He called his children at least three times a week. His children did come from the South to visit him at the hospice. His oldest son had to be forced to go. They saw him on Saturday and left on Sunday morning. On Monday afternoon at about 1:20, Ed died.

He wanted his obituary to say that he died of AIDS. He talked to me about it and also to his parents. However, they did not grant his last wish.

What have my experiences with Ed taught me?

I guess I am much more aware of the reality that we are all spiritual beings first. We happen to exist for a time, find ourselves in a physical body. Ed's life and death taught me that happiness can't be found with more alcohol or more food or more sex. Those things might gratify us for a time, but they will not ultimately satisfy us. We must look to our spirituality. Another general, overall thing he taught me was to *own* some of my own anger; to not be willing to swallow my anger, which is classic for priests. We are always nice. We get angry like everybody else, but because we're expected to always be nice, we don't express it. He also taught me to love and care for myself more.

What would I say to Ed if I could?

Compassion comes only when we discover the very one we were created to be. Sharing your spiritual journey to wholeness aided my resolving issues of misinformation, losses of control, and, of course, human loneliness. From the compassion of your very self, I began to seek my wholeness. Thank you for this gift.

Watching and being with you as the bonds of shame were loosened, I began my healing and homecoming. Every day my inner child misses your joy, laughter, and enthusiasm for life. Such life, which is your unique soul, can now sing, dance, and shout in ways not limited by flesh and bone.

—JOHN HESCHLE

☐ Ed died on July 8, 1991, at the age of 43. Says John Heschle of his former buddy, "I know it would please Ed very much to know he is a part of this project."

"I cried, thinking of my poor family. I'm going to die and rob my children of a mother. How will they get along? Who is going to care for my husband and children?"

—FROM THE JOURNAL OF JENNIFER FOLSOM
after learning that she was HIV-positive

"I thought only people who use drugs or are gay have AIDS. Not my kid."

—JUNE KENNEY
Jennifer's mother

In September 1990, June Kenney's daughter, Jennifer, age 29, died of AIDS. Six weeks later, so did her three-year-old granddaughter.

We did not know that Jen was sick. First of all, she got married to Doug. About a year later, they had Nicolette. There were no problems whatsoever with that pregnancy. Jennifer was very healthy. She used to walk five miles a day. After Niki was born, Jen used to work as a hairdresser and as a waitress.

Then they had another baby. After Angela was born in May 1987, Jennifer's health changed. She was tired and just didn't ever get back on her feet. The doctors couldn't find anything wrong and told us that sooner or later she'd come out of it. She didn't.

□ After being sent home, Jennifer's fatigue, diarrhea, night sweats, and other symptoms continued. She returned to the hospital for more tests—cancer, leukemia, lupus. They were all negative.

Then, one night back in their home, Jennifer and her husband, Doug, were watching television. There on the screen was U.S. Surgeon General C. Everett Koop. He spoke about a new disease.

The following morning, Jennifer drove to Burlington from her Duxbury, Vermont, home and went to the doctor. Three days later she was told she was HIV-positive.

> *"RAGE!!! I'm too young to die. I'm so confused; I have a dreaded disease that I know absolutely nothing about."*
>
> **—FROM JENNIFER'S JOURNAL**

When Doug said, "AIDS," my head reeled. Jennifer had tested positive, but Doug was negative. And I think that was a lot of his problem, because from then on he felt, Why *her?* Why not *me?*

It was very stressful. I mean, the bills were coming in. Jennifer wanted to go public with it. Doug didn't want her to. He was afraid people wouldn't come down to his garage to have their cars fixed because his wife had AIDS. So we told people that she had leukemia. I felt so bad lying. I had taught my kids to tell the truth. But we live in a small town, and we didn't know what would happen. We felt trapped.

☐ In May 1988, just after Angie's first birthday, Jennifer, Doug, and June found out that Angie also had tested positive for the AIDS virus. The family told their friends and neighbors that she had leukemia.

Eventually, in June 1989, at a weekend seminar conducted by Dr. Bernie Siegel, Jennifer took the microphone and announced, "My name is Jennifer Folsom, and I have AIDS."

"I want to tell you I am proud of the woman I married. You have grown so much. . . . You and I are raising two beautiful people, inside and out. You should be proud, too."

—DOUG'S NOTE TO JENNIFER
on their final wedding anniversary

☐ But, despite his obvious love for his wife and family, Doug Folsom could no longer endure the devastation of the disease. After four years of being on the wagon, Doug started to drink. Jennifer wrote in her journal, "My husband: Denial. Relapse of alcoholism. Guilt. No self-worth. No dealing with family life. Excuses. Fear."

Finally, in June 1990, Doug put a gun to his head and killed himself. Jennifer would later say, "He danced as long as he could."

At first, it was a terrible shock to Jennifer. It took her a while. But she told me that she was going to pick herself up by her boot straps and go on with life, and that she wanted to accomplish some things. And she did. She opened up an awful lot of people's eyes in Vermont.

☐ Six days after Doug shot himself, Jennifer went before her church and told the entire congregation the true nature of her illness. They responded by planning an event called "A Celebration of Life" for the Folsom Family Fund. The event, a sort of big community fair, was held in August. Local bands donated their music. Eighteen restaurants donated 10 percent of their earnings for the day. Shop owners donated T-shirts. They had pony rides, baseball dunks, clowns, and ice cream. And the entire community sang in the choir. The event raised eight thousand dollars that went into a fund for Niki's college education.

Jenny went to the community celebration and spoke. Everybody in the community came forward. Everybody, everybody. Nobody shunned her. We never got any nasty letters. We never got any hate letters. Niki was received very well in school.

Meanwhile, Angie was slowly going right through our fingers, and Jenny and I noticed it. Pediatric AZT was not available yet. She was dying right in front of us. She stopped walking. She was having severe headaches. She was not eating and was getting very thin. They put her on a feeding tube. It just didn't seem to be doing any good. She was having a lot of problems with infections. We took her down to Children's Hospital in Boston because of a sinus infection that she had developed. Again, the AZT was not available. Jen and I came home and I said, "You know, Jen, I can't stand this." She said, "Neither can I, Ma." We just looked at each other, and then we went out and got Jen's bottle of AZT and broke them into pieces, crushed them up, and put them in Angie's applesauce.

It seemed to help. It was funny because I took her into the doctor and he said, "She seems to be doing a little bit better. I don't know what you're doing, June, and I'm not going to ask you what you're doing. But whatever you're doing, keep doing it." I said,

"Thank you very much. I will." Jenny and I both did, because we had to do something. We were grasping at straws at that point. She was going to die, so why not? And it did help. A month after we did that, AZT became available for children.

☐ As Jennifer's condition worsened, June decided to quit her job to become a full-time caregiver to her daughter and granddaughter.

Jennifer was getting weaker and weaker. She couldn't eat. She had developed uterine cancer, and each month that she had her period, it took so much out of her. Until the very end, she would not take morphine because she knew what it did to her, and she had set two goals in her life. One was to attend the community fair. The other was to see her daughter, Niki, go to her first day of kindergarten.

And then the day came.

I went over at six o'clock in the morning. I got Niki up and dressed and then we went into Jen and said, "We're all ready to go to kindergarten." Jen said, "Mama, I have to *see* her go." I said, "No. You can say good-bye to her now." And she said, "No, damn it! I'm going to see her go!" She got out of bed, and I wrapped an afghan around her, put an umbrella over her, and carried her to the porch so that she could watch Niki walk down the path and board the school bus. That was on Tuesday. On Wednesday, Jen died. She passed away in my arms.

The day that Jen died, we packed up things and we moved Angela and Niki over to my house. Angie became my baby. Nobody was going to hurt her. I wanted Angie to live. I wanted them to find something, anything.

☐ Angie's condition continued to deteriorate before June's sleepless eyes. Finally, on a warm October night, June, no longer able to watch her daughter's baby writhe in pain, cried out to God in anguish: "I don't know what You're doing up there, but I wish You'd get down here and take Your baby!"

On that evening, a vision came to June. She remembers that she saw the hat Angie insisted on wearing whenever she left the house. It was made of blue canvas with pink bunny ears and a pushed-up visor. June says she ran to find the hat and placed it on Angie's head, and then she cradled her granddaughter in her arms and whispered, "Go now, baby, go. Go find Mommy.

"And she went. I put that hat on her head and she went."

What has gotten me through this?

Jenny and I had a very special relationship. We found something funny to laugh at every day.

And my belief in God helps me through it. There's one thing uppermost in my heart, that there is no *why* in God's plan. I just have to keep that in my mind.

And my husband and I are very, very close.

Also, I have been out speaking a lot to help other people under-stand this illness—to open their eyes that this is *here* and that it is only the tip of the iceberg. It is an issue, and we have to face it. The ones I really want to reach are the young people who are going to bring children into this world, because if they had walked in my shoes and held that baby the day she died the way I did, they wouldn't want to bring a child into the world who was going to die of AIDS.

It is important, and it's about time, that people stop treating people with AIDS like they're lepers. It's a disease. And it's not a gay disease. It's a people disease. I used to think that only people who used drugs or were gay had AIDS. Now I know better. Years ago I would have judged. I *did* judge. No more. How someone got AIDS doesn't matter. It matters that they have the disease and that we deal with them with love.

—JUNE KENNEY

☐ Before her death, Jennifer Folsom fought to educate the world about AIDS. She went to Congress to fight for further research about women with AIDS. She spoke out all over the United States. She crusaded for AIDS prevention, for the use of condoms, and for the practice of safe sex. Says her mother, "The day she died, the doctor said, 'I don't know if we really did that much for Jennifer—but Jennifer has done an awful lot for us.'"

Today June Kenney is continuing her daughter's legacy and continuing to fight to educate people about this disease. Says June, "I will speak almost anywhere anybody wants to hear me." In 1990, the state of Vermont named June Kenney its Mother of the Year.

Today Jennifer's other daughter, Nicolette Folsom, wears a gold *J* around her neck. And at school she has requested that her teachers and friends address her by a new name: Nicolette Jennifer Folsom.

I was told I was HIV-positive in 1984. I had ARC [AIDS-related complex] in late 1983, early 1984. I was paralyzed with nerve damage in my back and came down with bronchial pneumonia at the same time. I had shingles at the same time that were causing nerve problems in my chest and belly. When I was in the hospital, they also said that two of the discs in my back had deteriorated, and all of the nerve-pinching problems and stuff were being exaggerated by CMV.

I was paralyzed again in 1986—November 22, to be exact, when I collapsed in my bathroom. My two discs had deteriorated even more, and I wasn't getting neuroelectrical impulses to my brain from the lower part of my body. I was paralyzed for almost three months and was hospitalized.

There aren't words to describe it. Have you ever had hot needles stuck through your neck? Well, that's about as close to it as I can even think of. You get a shooting pain from the small of your back all the way up your spine and into several parts of your brain, including these incredible pinpoint things that happen on the left side of your head. You have no warning whatsoever. I collapsed in the post office today with a money bag from our store. The bag fell out of my hands, and the money rolled all over the place. I dropped my letters. I don't scream out when it happens. I do bite my tongue, and I get tears because it hurts so intensely.

I take a drug called Calmforte, which is a holistic, herbal medicine. I take three of these at a time when this happens, and my body starts to relax within 15 minutes.

I don't take antivirals. I don't care to pollute my body anymore. I know what AZT does to you. I know what DDI does to you. I know what Compound Q does to you. And I know what DDC [Dideoxycytidine] does to you. They are all highly toxic. AIDS activists and others pushed to have the drugs put on the market before they even finished the trials. And I'm not taking something that turned my best friend toxic in two weeks and killed him.

I did take prednisone for a year and three months. It's a steroid, a cortisone-derivative drug, and it messes you up. You're not supposed to be on it any longer than you are on AZT, which, some doctors say, is nine months. Finally I took myself off prednisone voluntarily, as I had done several years before with other more illicit drugs. I had gone sober three years before. I knew I had to get sober because it was killing me.

What would I say to other people who are HIV-infected?

I hate to sound really old-fashioned about this, but try not to put too many toxins in your body. I mean, we're already breathing polluted air. We're eating foods that have either been preserved or have high sugar content. Don't add extra things, things like crystal heroine. There's a whole new crowd coming up who loves LSD. Just like the old days. These guys are 21, 22, 23 years old. I tell them, "I took it for the first time in 1966. What the hell's wrong with you? *Don't* take it."

Keep your sense of humor, always, always. No matter what. I have not been depressed since the day I first went into the hospital.

On that day, lying in that bed, I resolved then and there—because I had almost died twice in that period—that I would never allow my mental faculties to weaken, no matter how much I deteriorated physically. But my sense of humor is the most important thing to me. I've laughed through two boyfriends, a boyfriend of six and a half years, and my best friend, all of whom died of AIDS. That's been four deaths in eight years.

I hate to dredge up clichés, but you get this incredible wellspring of strength that starts in you at some point and just builds and builds. Yes, you are vulnerable, but you think, "Well, I can handle this. I'm strong." It's degrading what you have to go through in the hospital. In the early days of AIDS, I was put in an isolation room. People had to put on gowns, masks, and gloves when they came in to confront me about all this. It was dehumanizing. I learned strength and more strength. When I went sober I had to have 100 percent strength. When I was told I had AIDS, I just had to summon up another 100 percent. I thought, "For God's sake, where can I get that from?" You'd be surprised.

What do I miss most?

Well, I stopped doing several sex acts that I was very fond of. You might underline that several times: fond of. Because, I'm a very visual person. Visually, to me, sex is probably the greatest joy I'll ever feel in my life. That and helping a woman friend give birth to a child.

I've changed in the last nine, ten years. I'm less angry than I was in the beginning. I'm also more resolved that something I'm unaware of could happen and that my life will go. And that I will not have completed what I wanted to do.

I want to complete everything. Life, people, animals, our relationship to the planet. I work in a bookstore so I can just gather it all in, like picking fruit off trees. I've always read. It's my escape. I tried drugs for a while. Those didn't work. I went back to reading. That's the only way I can go anywhere. I don't have enough money to go to the places I've read about. I've wanted to visit Australia, Scotland, Japan, China. I've read everything I possibly can about certain countries and cultures and their art and their lives because I love it. That's my travel.

What do I see when I look into the mirror?

Nothing. I don't look into mirrors. I just get up and thank God that the water boils for tea, that I still have gas, that I paid the bill. You know, the simple pleasures.

☐ Steven Morris, 39, is working as a bookstore manager in West Hollywood. His childhood ambition was to travel.

Eighteen years ago Joseph Camaya and Walter McWethy
lost contact with each other. Then, one day in 1988,
Walter telephoned his old friend and told him that he had
AIDS. At the time, Joseph was an AIDS volunteer and
buddy, and he welcomed Walter back into his life with
open arms and mind. Today their friendship has evolved
into a study in shared experience and mutual respect.

Walter is an activist, I know that. I also know that through some
of his activism he has stepped on a few toes and made enemies
during his journey with HIV and AIDS. From my training and education as a volunteer with Shanti [a Los Angeles AIDS service organiza-
tion], I knew the additional stress Walter took upon himself was
not in his best health interest. I wanted to educate him about the
stress he was taking on and what it could do to him. Through our
conversations I realized he was very well aware of this epidemic
he faced and of the sacrifices he was willing to make.

I've known Walter for over 20 years now. When I met him back in
the early '70s, he was in the Air Force, stationed in San Bernardino,
California. We were wild and crazy, as young men are in their early

20s. I noticed then that Walter, when wronged, stood up for his rights. He has more guts than I, I thought back then, and I admired his courage to challenge people and demand rights denied him.

Somehow I felt secure when Walter was around. He was like a lighthouse in a fogged-in harbor—always there for you and willing to help. Walter eventually married and had a little boy. Was he happy? I don't know. I had lost contact with him during those years. I do know that he loved children. Children were the thing that inspired him. I later learned that he had lost his wife and son in a car accident. Walter was devastated. He began to drink heavily and fell into drugs.

Eight years ago he hit bottom and decided to stop his self-destruction and join Alcoholics Anonymous. In memory of his boy, he created a character named Santa Mouse. That is, he put on a mouse costume with a Santa Claus coat and hat and visited orphanages and hospitals, giving his love and compassion to the less fortunate children in the community.

At about the same time, Walter began to get sick, and an HIV test proved that he was indeed infected. He then dove into this epidemic that was robbing us all of our brothers and sisters. He initiated contributions to a failing food bank, where others had been unable to get commitments, and helped it flourish. He involved himself in the local AIDS project as a spokesperson. And it was there that he experienced some political problems. He began to question procedures he felt were unnecessary and stressful to clients applying [to the organization] for assistance.

That's when I came into contact with Walter again. It had been about 15 years since I had seen him. He had contacted my brother and told him of his condition. My brother said, "Joe can help. He's worked with the AIDS project in Los Angeles. Give him a call." When I got Walter's phone call, I was very surprised and pleased.

But I asked myself, Why is he such a troublemaker? Why can't he just take care of himself and leave those people [at the local AIDS project] alone? Those people were giving of themselves, their time, compassion, and love in volunteering for the war against this epidemic. As a volunteer myself, I know firsthand some of the sacrifices we make to give of ourselves. I also know that with the stress of this work some of us can lose sight of our motives. But, certainly, they could do no wrong. So I would say to Walter, "You're marching *where?* Picketing *who?* Newspapers, radio, and television? *What* petition?"

Eventually, I *had* to know the cause of his rebellion. Walter explained. "Joe," he said, "I believe I have been treated improperly and that there were injustices against me, my brothers, and my sisters. Some of the procedures executed by this organization [the local AIDS project] seemed unnecessarily stressful for me. I looked around and saw many others too weak to speak up. I can and do, not only for myself, but for those who can't."

I began to see Walter differently. I know he isn't 100 percent right all the time, but who is? Yet, if he felt he was right, he went head-on, face-to-face. People on the other side of his crusade saw an enemy, a troublemaker, and couldn't see the hero I now visualized. He stood up for the weak and meek. He spoke his words and the words they couldn't.

This crusade has taken its toll on Walter. Santa Mouse is now retired. Have the children lost? His activism is quiet now. Have our brothers and sisters lost? I know there will be others to take Walter's place when he's gone. Now I will look at them in a completely different light.

Have I changed because of my ongoing journey with Walter? I'm no longer afraid to say what's on my mind. I'm no longer tolerant of those who would deny me my rights as a human being. I stand up and speak out for my rights and for the rights of others who are either too afraid or too weak.

I will also try to put on this damn mouse costume . . . except the shoes seem too big.

—JOSEPH CAMAYA

I lost my wife and son eight years ago in a car accident, right before I tested HIV-positive.

We can go back 10 years in determining that there was something definitely wrong. I had had swollen glands two years prior to losing my wife and son. The surgeons kept on turning down my request for a biopsy of the glands of the neck because it was in the central nerve area. They were afraid that if they cut, they might do some damage.

After losing my wife and my son, I fell into the dilemma of destroying myself with alcohol and drugs. I didn't even care about life. I didn't even know that I was a beautiful person—until I got sick.

I had my first attack of pneumocystis in 1984. I've had pneumocystis now three times. I can't keep my nutrition down. They're tube feeding me. It's either go into the hospital or stay home with an IV pole. Now I'm battling tuberculosis. I had to have two stomach surgeries to determine whether or not I had it. Now the tuberculosis has gotten into my intestines and is eating them away. It's like a stomach monster on a daily routine. That's why I can't hold down a lot of food. It either comes up or goes out. I don't have a desire to eat anymore. Everything I put in me, whether it's fluid or solid food, hurts. It's very painful.

I've been hurt by my real family. Rejected. Even though I came close to death three times this year, my family still will not come near me. They have a fear of AIDS, of coming in contact with AIDS. They're afraid. I can't kiss them. I can't hug them. I have a sister who lives close by and she's never been to my home. My own mother is afraid to hug me.

The only time that I hear from my real family is if I pick up the phone and call them or write to them. I still don't give up. I keep trying.

But that's OK. I continue to go to the hospital to visit my brothers and sisters with AIDS or cancer every Easter and every Christmas. At Christmastime I make up care packages; at Easter I make Easter baskets and take them flowers. I have a lot of people who support me in helping me with my care packages.

And I met a very special woman eight years ago, when I was first diagnosed. She has cancer. Her name is Betty Flanagan. Betty took me by the hand, like a mother. Betty's my best friend today. She's 68 years old. I have to take my hat off to Betty for her experiences of living with and dealing with cancer.

Today my family is made up of my friends. I have many, many people out there who support me. When I say I'm going into the hospital, they ask how high they should jump. I'm very grateful for my friends like Joe Camaya. Joe and I have known each other for 20 years, and we go all the way back to our early 20s, you know, when young men will be wild and crazy.

I guess I would say that I'm probably more gay than bisexual. But I don't even know what that means. I haven't had sex in a long time—and I care not. All I want are the hugs and the kisses and to know that tomorrow will be a better day if you just believe.

How did I change my life?

I decided I was going to live a better life. I have found a new God, a God I never knew was there. He is a God that has provided me with much more than monetary values; He has provided me with values of love.

I want to help my brothers and sisters who are suffering out there, who don't understand what's going on. I have a lot to give them. I have a lot to share with them about how I've changed my life the last eight years. Every time I'm admitted to a hospital for AIDS, I put my illness aside for someone else and I try to get them to understand how I'm fighting it. I'm a brother of love, a brother of peace. All I want to see is peace in the world and us helping each other, instead of all this fighting and politics and money-hungry people.

If you cannot help your fellow brother and sister out there, you're no good. When my brothers and sisters are too afraid or too weak to stand up for their rights, I'm not. I'm tired of people crying and doing nothing.

Nobody out there can hurt us just because we're sick.

Can't we help each other?

—WALTER McWETHY

☐ Walter McWethy, formerly and belovedly known as "Santa Mouse," is 37 years old. He has been living with HIV for nine years.

84

My ex-husband was HIV-positive. When he got his diagnosis in 1986, we had been married for about three and a half years and had been together for five and a half years. He was trying to get back into the military, and they did an HIV test on him without his knowledge. Then they sent him a letter in the mail that he had AIDS, because in 1986, that's what they were telling people who tested positive.

After his diagnosis, we did not practice safe sex. We should have. I just assumed that since he was [HIV-positive], I was. The doctor took two months to figure out what was wrong with me. I was like, "Well, what's wrong? What's wrong with me? I'm tired. I keep running these fevers." It was, for me, more of a relief to know that they had finally come up with a diagnosis.

My husband didn't do anything about his HIV for almost two years after his diagnosis. When he finally did go see a doctor, his T-cell count was 64, and we went into a major panic. All my energies were more or less concentrated on him. It was amazingly stressful to try to keep everything normal, so to speak. We hid it from my mom, who was ill. Then we found out that his sister, his younger sister, had AIDS. She eventually died less than a year after my diagnosis. She was 32.

My husband's the one who left. I think he felt very guilty. I just don't think he could handle it. I, on the other hand, don't know if I was handling it very well, either. I know it brought a definite strain into our relationship. And it really affected my teenage daughter. She stopped going to school and started having a whole lot of psychological problems.

I didn't get through my husband's leaving well at all. My mom had just died, maybe four months prior to that, not knowing my status.

Initially, I refused to be on AZT. I've now been on it for a year. I'm also on Bactrim, and I take Chinese herbs and do acupuncture.

Now my ex-husband has full-blown AIDS. My stepkids deal with it by being totally in denial. My daughter is in denial too, but at least she's doing little things like trying to get more information.

How have I gotten through this?

I'm in a 12-step program, I was very active with that, on the board of directors, but I was getting tired of censoring my conversations. So I talked it over with my therapist and decided that I would come out and say I was HIV-positive at the next meeting. So I stood at the podium and told my story, and of the 150 people there, I'd say there were five who were just shocked and appalled. Everyone else was very loving and supportive. One lady came up to me and said, "Do I have an organization for you!" She brought me to Shanti and introduced me to the people there.

Then I took the Plus seminar [sponsored by Shanti] and decided that since I was healthy, I needed to let people know that you *can* live with this disease, that everyone is not shriveled up and dying. The only pictures that I had ever seen of people with AIDS were of gay white men who were thin and emaciated and just on their last legs. To me, that was so scary. I just want people to know that, first of all, heterosexuals *do* get this disease. And that we have lives, and we have children, and we plan futures, and we live with this disease.

Now I'm a volunteer at Shanti. It started out as one day a week, and now it's extended to three.

What would I say to others?

This is not a death sentence. Plan your future. Because you *do* have a future. For me, that's the most important thing, to know that I do have a future. There was a time when I couldn't plan past a year. Hopefully, my daughter is going away to college in a few weeks. And you know, it has never crossed my mind one time that I will not be at her graduation.

HIV has allowed me to be more vocal. It has allowed me to look at myself and know that I can make a difference. I'm not as shy as I used to be in most situations. I think I'm more outgoing. You know what? I'm happier than I've ever been.

I know it sounds weird. When I tell people that, they go, "Excuse me?" But I am happier than I've ever been. I'm helping people. I'm making a difference by being an example. I think I'm making a positive statement. And I'm living my life. I'm walking the walk and talking the talk. I'm clean, I'm sober, I'm abstinent. I've got a beautiful daughter and I've got a dog that I love.

—PATRICIA GRIFFIN

☐ Patricia Griffin is 40 years old. She tested HIV-positive on December 23, 1987. As of this writing she is still relatively healthy and is entertaining the possibility of having another relationship. Says Patricia, "Sure, if the right person comes along, I'd be open to getting married again."

❑   ❑

I walked into a classroom at LACC [Los Angeles City College] this
fall. I had already graduated from there, *magna cum laude,* number
two in a class of 650. I was studying psychology. Anyway, I went
back and walked into a classroom this fall. It was a political-science
class. The first day, the professor made an announcement that if
you were late for class, you were out of there, unless you had a
doctor's excuse. The second time the class met, I had just come
from a pentamidine treatment that had run a little late, so I walked
into the class half an hour late. When I did, the professor said in
front of the whole room that I was dismissed from the class. I said,
"Well, I was at the doctor and I have a doctor's excuse. You said
that would be acceptable." And as I went to hand him the excuse
he commented that I didn't look sick to him. I said, "Well, I'm a
person with AIDS." He said he wished that I hadn't told him that.
Then I said, "Why?" He said that he didn't want to handle my papers
because they don't know everything there is to know about AIDS.

That was the first time in almost five years of living with AIDS
that I ever, ever, ever felt dirty, ashamed, defenseless. Most of the
other students, quite frankly, were very much on his side.

It went back and forth for a while, and then he said that he didn't know if he wanted me in his class and that I didn't have a choice in the matter. I said, "I'm enrolled in the class legitimately, and I am legally protected to be here." He responded by saying that he might have to see me in court.

Then I said, "Well, listen, there's only three ways of transmission. I'm not having unsafe sex with you, we're not sharing needles, and I'm not your mother, you're not my fetus, so I wouldn't be worried about it." He flipped out.

Anyway, there was a break, after which he came back to me and said that he was sorry if he had embarrassed me, but that I was the one who said I had AIDS. I said, "I'm not embarrassed about my illness, and that's not the issue. The issue is your comments about my staying in the class." He repeated that he didn't know if he was going to let me stay in the class and that he'd let me know the following week.

The message that he sent to all the other students, who were not really AIDS savvy, was that, well, maybe we can get AIDS from him. His abuse of responsibility is unconscionable in 1991, in a classroom, in a school that's publicly funded.

I then went to Affirmative Action to file a discrimination claim against him. They finally ruled against me, saying that the professor made these statements out of ignorance and therefore they were not mal-intended, nor did they come from a place of hatred. Anyway, it's an ongoing thing. Of course, we're appealing it.

I've been HIV-positive at least since 1983. On December 23, 1986, I was given an ARC diagnosis. I've been on AZT for a very long time, three years. I was one of the first people on it. Initially, it was dreadful. You know, 1,200 milligrams a day. I was sick as a dog and all of that. But once I got over that hump, probably after the second month, the dosages were decreased, and it was OK. I'm not attributing it exclusively to AZT, I don't want to do that, but I'm very sure that it has been a major part of my hanging around as long as I have.

When I was diagnosed with ARC, I was given a six-month prognosis. But the six months came and went, and it didn't happen. So at some point I thought, well, it isn't happening, I might as well get on with my life. And so that's what I did. I got clean and sober. And then what happened, one of the things that changed my life completely, was that I fell in love. And I'm still with the same man today.

When people say that AIDS changed their lives, I hate that. Yeah, it changed my life. And yes, it's a learning experience. But it's not a change I wanted, nor is it an experience that I cared to learn firsthand. Is it a change I wanted? Or something that I'm grateful about? Absolutely not. No way. I would have much rather learned about it from reading a book, although I know that the lesson wouldn't have been the same. It's a horror. This is a horrible disease.

What lessons have I learned from having AIDS?

It's something I knew before AIDS, actually. I've lived my whole life with honesty being number one. I also believe in developing profound love with people. If it means losing people along the way, that's fine. But develop loving relationships everywhere you go in your life. And the only way I believe you can do that is through honesty. And so if you come from a place of honesty and have loving relationships, then AIDS doesn't mean shit.

What would I say to other people?

Look at everything that's out there. But ultimately, listen to your heart. I believed all my life that we always know the answer. That's the thing. We always know the answers for us. We know what's right. And all we have to do is listen to ourselves.

90

And this is really important: If you don't have a family, make one. Don't whine about it. Don't complain about it. Make one. Do it.

—WAYNE KARR

☐ Wayne Karr, 37, has been something of an activist since childhood. Says he, "I was driving a tractor in drag when I was 10 years old. They didn't like it." As an adult AIDS activist, Wayne once went on a 10-day outdoor hunger strike to force the Food and Drug Administration to make AIDS-related drugs more accessible to those who need them.

As for his fight against his former professor at LACC, Wayne promises, "If I've got to go to my grave on this one, I will."

I've spent 18 years, 9 to 10 months of every year, on a bicycle. I lived on my bicycle. I would bicycle up to the Arctic Circle. I would bicycle everywhere. I had a goal to be the man who knew the continent. By the time I was in my 80s, I wanted to have known all of North America like no other living human being.

For 20 years I made my living by painting very elaborate stenciled ceilings in Victorian houses. But mostly I traveled. Every day I was 80 miles away from where I was the day before. I went 240,000 miles. I crossed the United States and Canada 23 times.

I was in Saratoga Springs, working in a little hotel in October, November of 1990, when I got this diarrhea. The doctor I went to there misdiagnosed me. He gave me Lomotil, a topical treatment for diarrhea, and that did end the symptoms. I thought it had gone away. Then I started bicycling back to the West Coast in December, and by the end of the month I got very sick. So I got on a train and went to San Francisco, moved in with a friend, and started trying to get a doctor, because by then *I knew*, you know?

I was diagnosed with cryptosporidiosis and AIDS in March 1991. They put me on AZT with an accelerated dosage, starting with one a day, until I was finally taking five a day. Initially, I tolerated it very well, but I only lasted for seven or eight months on it. Now I'm on DDI, which has been a really good treatment for me.

I had resisted getting tested for years. I just didn't want to know. I felt like I was immune. Athleticism is a very deceptive thing. If you really utilize your body physically—and I don't mean for one hour but for six and seven hours a day, for months and years—it can lead to abuses in your personality. You feel very powerful. You have a lot of energy. Things don't bother you. My history before this happened was that I wasn't a drug user or drinker or any of that. I'd go on binges. I'd hit a city and I'd just get plastered. Then I wouldn't drink for six months. And I would have sex with people and not really take precautions. I felt immune.

How has my life changed?

I no longer live on my bike. That's the big one. And for almost a year, I didn't do any painting. I felt very sad about not being able to bike. I've done short trips, like up the coast for 200 miles, but I get very exhausted after about 30 or 40 miles. I had to really give it up.

One of my favorite sayings when I used to travel by bicycle all the time was "no tragedy, no tale." When I first got sick, there had been a lot of periods of depression and everything. And I was stuck in bed. But from my bed, really sick and scared shitless, I contacted all the [support] services and started to sign up for them. My doctor directed me. She said, "You have AIDS, and this is what you do." She gave me lists of all these social organizations, social security income, and all that. During the first couple of months, I started to keep a list, meant to be funny, of all the positive things that have come out of this. They include:

- Free hot meals delivered
  [Project Open Hand]
- Free pedicure every 12 weeks
  [Pacific Coast Hospital Podiatry Clinic]
- I no longer have to worry about:
  a heart attack
  the ecological collapse
  nuclear war
- Free time [I'm retired]
- No need to diet

I wanted to get an apartment, but the problem was that the SSI money was not enough to rent an apartment in San Francisco. So the first thing I did was to go around to all these churches, about 25 of them, and ask to see the minister. I told them that I wanted to paint a church because I wanted to do something really wonderful and meaningful for my last major project. I told them that I was a person with AIDS and that what I wanted for this was an apartment to live in, because I did not have enough money from SSI to get an apartment.

Eventually, I found a church. The First Presbyterian. They built an apartment for me in a parishioner's basement and gave me a budget for the flooring and everything. It was really fun. I designed an apartment that was a good apartment to have AIDS in. Everything is moppable and washable. And I'm painting the church, and that makes me feel quite happy. I enjoy doing that a great deal. I figure I'm running a bargain with God. I'm painting His, or Her, house, and He or She had better be nice to me. The longer I'm around, the more that church gets painted.

It's almost getting exciting. I've never lived this way. I've got my first apartment I've ever had in my whole life. I absolutely love it. You know what I mean?

—*LARRY BOYCE*

☐ Larry Boyce is 45 years old. His childhood ambition was to be an astronomer, a goal he never realized. Still, his nighttime travels via bicycle provided him with something of an education. Says Larry, "I know my night sky very well."

What I Have

By Marc Wagenheim

I've just turned 34, and I've got things in my life that I never imagined I'd have. I have doctors—an internist, an infectious-disease gastroenterologist, a radiologist, an oncologist/hematologist—a home health-care nurse, a Monday-afternoon support group, a hospital I've spent so much time in that I know which floor and wing to ask for. I have a basket of pills I keep at my bedside and take throughout the day which includes medication that costs hundreds of dollars. I have a catheter that is inserted in the right side of my chest, through which I infuse a nutritional supplement for nine hours each night. To accompany the catheter and the infusion process, I have a cart full of medical supplies—tubing, syringes, needles, clamps, et cetera. I have a remarkable creative-writing group that meets on Saturday mornings. If you haven't guessed by now, I have AIDS.

I have people in my life who love me and care for me and support me. I have a special person who'll hold me at night sometimes when my temperature soars and the chills invade my body. I have a mother who loves me and believes in keeping our lives separate, yet who's always there when I need her to work her mother's magic. I have some friends I really don't talk to anymore, maybe because they're scared of the sadness; maybe because they're just scared.

I have a golden retriever I've had since he was just a fluff ball whom I adore and who will be 10 years old this summer. I have a sick sense of humor and tell people that he and I have the same life expectancy, though his blood work looks a lot better than mine.

I have a comfortable, warm, Spanish-style house that often consoles me and gives me a place to which I cherish returning. I have "things"—objects and knickknacks and souvenirs of a life that mean something but also mean less.

I have times when I'm very brave and strong and manage to climb out of a seemingly bottomless pit, and I have times when I'm very afraid.

☐ After battling with AIDS for five and a half years, and not long after he wrote "What I Have," Marc Wagenheim died on October 28, 1991. He left behind, among others, his lover of 10 years, Mark Winsten. "What I Have," an eloquent expression that speaks volumes, was written by Marc for his creative-writing group. One of his childhood ambitions was to become a writer.

97

I donated blood to the Red Cross every six months. I donated in 1984. The blood was rejected, and it came back in 1985. I got a registered letter on my birthday, February 10, 1985. It said that I was HIV-positive.

I didn't consider myself to be in a high-risk group. I was in a monogamous relationship. I had a boyfriend. I don't know whether he was bisexual or whether he was a drug user. There was a possibility of both. He was a big bullshitter. I had to get him out of my life. He tested positive, too. I know that at some point after me he had a wife and a kid. He was a bastard, a real bastard.

What would I say to other women who are HIV-positive?

I've met men by putting ads in the paper that state I'm HIV-positive. And every time I've placed an ad, there are always a million responses and always some pretty nice people. That's how I met this boyfriend I have now. He's HIV-negative. Most of them who answered the ads were negative.

And I would say to women who think that it's not going to happen to them: It happened to me. Women in our society are afraid that if they tell someone to wear a condom, the man's going to leave them. Just use condoms.

What have I learned?

I finally figured out that I wasn't living my life. I was, you know, afraid of dying, so I wasn't able to live. Now I'm starting to live. In the last year, I've started to live. I've bought a new car. I've got a boyfriend in a relationship that's committed. I've got everything I want, every single thing I've ever wanted. I'm painting. I'm dealing with my family better, partly because of therapy and partly because of the HIV. I'm not really responsible with money. I don't save money very well. But I think at this point, *Why the hell should I?*

—MARY KATHERINE

☐ Mary Katherine is 34 years old. As of this writing she is still healthy and still working as an office manager and as an artist.

In 1987 I got involved with Study 016, which was being run by the federal government. The purpose of the study was to determine what dosage of AZT was appropriate, or if any dosage was appropriate. This was a time when AZT was so brand-new that nobody knew what it was. Seven hundred thirty of us across the country volunteered for the test. And the one thing our study proved was that early intervention with AZT slowed down the transition from HIV to AIDS. At the end of the study, I think there were only 18 or 20 of us who had developed AIDS.

As of September 17, 1991, I have an AIDS diagnosis: Kaposi's sarcoma. I tested HIV-positive Thanksgiving week of 1987. I'm still on AZT. I also maintain a regime of spirulina, about 8 to 12 tablets a day, and garlic pills, 4 a day.

Since September I have had a very aggressive doctor who has treated each KS lesion independently with surface injections of—I think it was Velban, which kills each KS site within a matter of days to weeks. I've had them on my legs and thighs and arms, a couple on my neck and face, and a couple on my chest. They just started popping out all over. This week at the doctor was the first week that we had no lesions to treat.

There are two different groups I'm involved with. One is a support group at the Hollywood Presbyterian Church run by a heterosexual, non-HIV man who is a deacon of the church, and a young lady who is a heterosexual, non-HIV person as well. We have a tendency to forget they're not HIV-infected and that they aren't gay. Anyway, they are just two of the most wonderful people in the world. And I've developed a lot spiritually by attending this support group for the last three years.

And then, through Being Alive, there's one support group I go to on Friday nights which is a really strong, rowdy, raucous group. We have a lot of fun and get a lot of education and an exchange of information and ideas there.

After I retired from my job as a litigation secretary (it was extremely stressful) I was going absolutely stir-crazy here in the house. So I called Being Alive and told them I needed to *do* something. They said, "Get down here and train to be a volunteer." I've been there ever since. I've been watering the gardens at the new facility, I do peer counseling on the telephone, and, oh God, I've handled shovels and brooms and set up banquet tables and stuff. If I see something that needs doing, I pick it up and do it.

Then I became involved in a service called Connect. The original objective of it was to set up a dating service in Los Angeles for HIV-involved people—whether heterosexual, bisexual, gay, male, or female. I take the phone calls as they come in and send out application forms to people who want them. I might add it's a really reasonable service. The cost to each person is either a self-addressed stamped envelope or a one-dollar donation, and that's it.

For the last 6, 8, 10 years, the fear has been so prevalent that most HIV-involved people were convinced they could never have another relationship. Now, in the last year or two, with the improvement of the medications and protocols, they're discovering that,

Hey, we're liable to end up little old ladies and bag men if we don't do something about it. And now it's not impossible to reach out to somebody and have a relationship without being terrified. It's inevitable. We are all going to die. The only difference is that some of us have a better notion of when.

☐ Ted Mischuk is 49 years old. When asked what gets him through each day, Ted responded, "When I wake up in the morning, I say to myself, Well, I'm alive. And I go with that."

I was diagnosed with ARC in 1982. I had low helper cells, warts that wouldn't go away, candidiasis on my tongue, hepatitis, CMV, mononucleosis, pneumonia, herpes, and shingles, but I didn't have any of the diseases defined by the Centers for Disease Control that qualified me for an AIDS diagnosis. They hadn't even discovered the virus yet. They didn't discover the virus until after I was diagnosed with full-blown AIDS in 1984. In April of 1984 I was diagnosed with Kaposi's sarcoma and lymphoma.

In 1985 I was patient number one on the first antiviral drug they tried against AIDS. The drug was suramin, which I took for 39 weeks, one gram per week. Within six weeks, my KS lesions had completely disappeared. On May 30, 1985, Dr. Alexander Levine, my doctor, called me to say that both of my cancers were within complete remission. They had suppressed the virus. I continued on the drug until the end of the year, but it proved to be very toxic. They had put 90 other people on the drug around the country, and it killed a number of them. The others died from the progression of the disease itself. As for me, I suffered adrenal deficiency, blindness, and some muscular damage. I also lost all my hair, was paralyzed on the left side of my body, and had terrible peripheral neuropathy. After I got off the drug, all that cleared up within about four months. I began to get better in March of 1986, and I haven't been sick with anything worse than the flu since them.

The virus is dormant, I guess. The drug has been out of my system for five or six years. Apparently, there are a lot of people who are walking around HIV-positive but the virus isn't doing anything. I seem to have returned to that state.

In fact, I believe that I've become healthier since I was diagnosed. And that's due to my intentionally working on taking responsibility for my own life, as well as laughing a lot, enjoying life, nurturing myself, and just doing things that are good for me. Not that I wasn't doing these things before, but I think now I do them more intentionally and more intensively.

There's nobody who understands an alcoholic like another alcoholic. Similarly, there's nobody who quite understands what it's like to be diagnosed and to live with HIV and AIDS like someone else who's been diagnosed with it. When I walk into the hospital room of somebody who's just been diagnosed and say, "Hi, my name's Steve Pieters and I've had this for nine years and I'm doing fine," the look, the transformation that happens on that person's face is incredible. Usually, people are quite despairing at that point, and then somebody walks in, healthy, robust, and pumping iron, and they go, "Oh, God! Maybe I can do it too." So, that's really helpful to other people, and I couldn't do that if I hadn't gone through it myself.

I think volunteer work, *getting outside yourself,* is vital to health.

When I was a kid, I was sent to summer camp, and I was very homesick. My grandmother wrote me a letter that said, "Find yourself another little boy who's homesick and see if the two of you can't help each other be not so homesick." And I found that worked, so all my life I've sought out opportunities to be of service. When

104

I was diagnosed, I wasn't working because I was too sick, and I had a lot of time on my hands. I wasn't so sick that I couldn't get out of the house and do *something*. I mean, being sick for years at a time is boring!

So I got involved over at AIDS Project Los Angeles back in 1984. I thought volunteer work would do me some good, and I could decide how many hours I was going to put in. I was the 80th client at APLA, and they didn't have a lot of clergy who were clients, so they put me to work on the phones and stuff. After about a year, they invited me to be on the board of directors, where I served for five and a half years before I was named to the board of governors.

My faith has helped a lot. I very much believe that God is my partner in fighting this, and cocreator of my wellness. During the darkest part of my illness, I could always find solace in reciting prayers, scripture passages, and when I was able to get to a piano, singing hymns. I remember thinking that if God is greater than the death of Jesus, then God is greater than AIDS.

When I went into the ministry [in 1979], I certainly didn't think I would be dealing quite so intensively with people my own age dying. I couldn't have imagined that. If anything, AIDS has deepened my faith. It's helped me realize that I can do a lot more than I thought I could. It's really made me a lot more confident in God. I think that it has intensified everything. I would say that I don't believe in a God who's a punishing God. I believe that God loves us. He loves us so much that sometimes we can't even understand or accept it. I think the challenge is to accept the fact that we are loved. It's easier sometimes to feel like we're being punished. But I try to get people to consider the question of why good people suffer. Why do bad things happen to good people? I point out that there are a lot of good people before them who have had bad things happen to them.

When I was diagnosed, one of the things that really hit my gut was that I was going to die without ever having been in a relationship. I was told that I had eight months, that I wouldn't live to see 1985, and I couldn't conceive of anybody being interested in someone with AIDS anyway. I had a chaplain who said, "Oh, yes, there's somebody for everybody." I went, "Right." But after I managed to outlive the doctor's expectancy, a man whom I had been friends with back in Hartford, Connecticut, a pastor there, offered to move in with me as my lover. I was starting with the suramin treatments at the time and was really excited and happy about it all. He moved in and we were happy—for about three weeks. It took about five months for him to leave. Since then, I've dated, but very occasionally.

What would I say to other people with AIDS?

Well, I think the first thing is to decide whether you really want to live. And if you want to live, then you have to believe in the possibility of getting well or, at the very least, of living with this, of coming to peace with the virus and learning to battle individual opportunistic infections as they come up with everything you've got. But I think the most important thing is having the right attitude, believing in the possibility of longtime survival and doing everything you can to make sure that happens. Educate yourself. Read as much as possible and pick out that which seems to make sense to you in terms of creating the conditions for wellness in your body.

This disease is not 100 percent fatal. *I'm living proof!*

—STEPHEN PIETERS

☐ Stephen Pieters, 39, is the field director of AIDS ministry for the Universal Fellowship of Metropolitan Community Churches. He lectures and tours around the world, spreading his messages of faith, hope, and longtime survival in the face of AIDS.

Ida Hoffman tested HIV-positive in February 1987. At the same time, her husband, Arthur, also tested positive. Ida took care of Arthur until his death in 1989.

When I met Arthur in 1974, he was everything that I wanted—regardless of what he had done with his life, regardless that he was an active drug user. He was the type of man I had always wanted for myself. I didn't want to be rich. I didn't want to have a fine home or car. I just wanted to take one day at a time and have his love and respect. He was the love of my life.

I found out I was a carrier of the AIDS virus in February 1987 when my husband found out that he was a carrier, but I didn't do anything about it. In August of 1988 my husband started getting very sick.

The doctor didn't put us on any medication. He didn't treat my husband for AIDS. My husband was suffering from pains in his lungs. The doctor said that Arthur had chest pains and treated him only for that. Now, as I read and learn, I think the pains were due to tuberculosis. You know, being a carrier of the AIDS virus, you have to be tested for TB every year.

We stopped going to that doctor, who no longer wanted to treat Arthur because he didn't know what he was treating him for.

In September Arthur went to the infectious-disease clinic here in New Jersey, where they told him he had cryptococcal meningitis. And that he had AIDS.

He remained in the hospital for nine months. While there, he went into shock and had a stroke. When he had this stroke he could not move his arms. He could not move his legs. He could not talk. He'd stay in a chair, and all he would do all day was holler. I was there every day, all day. I'd give him physical therapy, help him move his arms and legs, and help him talk. About three or four months later he started moving his hands and started feeding himself. Finally, he was discharged and came home, but all of a sudden he started getting sick again.

The lives of people with AIDS are being shortchanged because we're dealing with doctors who don't know what they're doing. My husband dealt with a doctor who just did not know anything about AZT. My husband didn't find out anything about AZT until 1988, but the doctors didn't give it to him, because they thought he was too sick and that it would give him side effects. I kept telling them to put him on AZT. They should have put him on AZT, but they didn't.

We lived together for 15 years. We weren't married, but we were living in common law. We got married just before Arthur's death. The hospital didn't feel that he was competent to make up his mind about the marriage, and I had to go through a legal battle with the hospital and with his family. They finally determined that he *was* competent. And he wanted to come home. So he came home and we got married. He died on November 1, 1989.

What would I say to other people?

I would suggest to people that if you love your common-law spouse, get married. Get married as soon as possible. Because if you don't, you're going to go through [legal] hell. And by all means, if you can't get married, try to get power of attorney.

I learned about family members. You need their support. Once you're a carrier and you're sick, if you don't have moral support from family or from people who care, you can automatically just give up. I do have a few enemies that I wish badness to. I know I shouldn't. But I do.

I also learned that your immune system is the most important thing and that if you are sick, you don't want to be homeless. You don't want to be out here in these streets breathing in this pollution. I'm trying to start a shelter for the homeless in New Jersey who are carriers of the HIV virus. Once they leave the hospital, they don't have any family members, anyone who loves them.

Doctors. You can't put any trust in them; that's what I've learned. Always get a second opinion.

There's so much we can do—and have to stop doing. We have to stop doing the things we used to do. Arthur and I stopped doing drugs in 1988 when he got real sick. We have to do the things that are right to keep us alive for as long as possible.

All the nurses in the hospital were telling me, "Ida, you'd better get to the clinic. You know you're a candidate. You'd better get on AZT." But I was too concerned about my husband's illness to worry about myself. I finally started going to the clinic in June 1988 and got myself on AZT.

I talk to God every day and just ask Him to keep me strong, to give me the strength to go on one more day, because I know that it's not promised to me. What I want most of all, though, is to die like my husband, with strength and dignity, because all through his illness, I'd never seen him so strong, so one hell of a man.

Sometimes I wake up and look in the mirror and say, "God, am I waking up? Do I have to wake up?" I know it's not right. I know, well, I have God and I shouldn't feel this way. And I know that my husband doesn't want me to feel this way. He wants me to go on and keep on trying from day to day. And that's what I'm doing.

—IDA HOFFMAN

☐ Ida Hoffman is 45 years old. Before testing HIV-positive, she worked as a nurse's assistant.

Her childhood dream was "to meet a man like my husband."

> *"It is with very heavy heart that I announce that effective immediately I must leave my medical practice. I have personally chosen to notify certain patients of my situation. It will not be possible to notify everyone.*
>
> *"Please share this information with any fellow patient who may not receive it."*
>
> **—DR. DON HAGAN**
> from a letter sent to his
> patients in March 1988

*B*eing a doctor, I've seen 20 or 30 people die with AIDS. Before, I couldn't imagine how they were feeling.

I went to a friend of mine who was a doctor. When he couldn't explain why I was having the constant headaches that I had been having for months, I went to get tested anonymously at a gay and lesbian clinic in Long Beach. My lover, Drew, doesn't handle things like this well. He would rather put a movie in the VCR than deal with AIDS, so I waited for him to leave town on a business trip, and I decided to have the test done.

I was called into this little room and sat down at a plain wooden table. When the person walked in the door, I interpreted in his face that the test was positive. It was.

It was a devastating moment, because it confirmed my worst fears. In the matter of a few seconds, all of the possible scenarios went flashing through my mind. What happens to my job? What happens to my income? What happens to Drew? How am I going to tell Drew this? We're one and a half years into a wonderful relationship, and what if he's positive? What if I've infected him? All of those things.

I have told lots of people that they have cancer, they have leukemia. I've told people they had AIDS. But for it to be personalized was very different.

I got home and I cried.

I met Drew in New Orleans—we are both from there—and when I told him, we cried in each other's arms. I knew that he was the special lifemate for me. I was afraid that maybe I had infected him or that he would leave. Drew got tested, and he was HIV-positive, too. But we both feel we were infected long before we became involved, and we do practice safe sex.

Soon after I was diagnosed, I started taking AZT, which had no side effects on me at all. I did real well with it for about a year and a half, and than I started getting headaches 24 hours a day and intestinal problems. In February 1988 I decided to retire 20 years earlier than I had planned. Some people want to work until they die, but I wanted to spend some quality time with my lover while I was still well enough to enjoy life. Drew twisted my arm and got me to take scuba-diving lessons, and I got certified! We went scuba diving a lot until recently. Now I'm just not well enough to go.

I stayed on AZT for four years. In May of 1990 I started taking a combination of AZT and DDI. By May of 1991 I was having reactions to the DDI including neuropathy so bad in my legs and my toes that I had to stop taking it. Then I started DDC with AZT, but I was having a lot of problems with the DDC, so I went off it. I didn't take anything for a while but Bactrim to prevent pneumocystis.

Through this entire ordeal I haven't had any hospitalizations with any major illnesses. I've been very lucky in that respect. Now I'm back on DDI, and I'm tolerating it better than I did the first time. During June and July of 1991 I was so sick, the sickest I have ever been since I was diagnosed in 1986. I had been having continuous fevers and night sweats every night. Some nights I soaked not only the sheets but even the mattress cover. Because of the night sweats and fevers, I had prolonged loss of appetite and was always tired. My sleep patterns were thrown out of whack. I lost 20 pounds. I am six-foot-three and weigh 180 pounds. Before I got sick, my weight was 200 pounds, and I worked out four days a week. I was very proud of my body. Now I'm tall and very skinny. Since August I've been back on the DDI, and I'm feeling much better.

Drew and I are getting ready to spend six weeks in the French quarter in New Orleans. We have an apartment there. We are taking our two dogs and driving there this weekend. My family is there, and so is Drew's. We are very lucky. We both have the support of our families.

I'm very realistic about this disease, and I don't have a problem with dying, but I really wonder about my future. I wonder if I will live in horrible pain, and if so, should I endure the pain? I know I have lived a very rich and full life. There aren't many things I wanted to do that I haven't done, and that is very comforting to me and to Drew. One of the only things people with AIDS never lose control of is the choice of how you want to live or die with this disease.

It's a very personal choice, but it is your choice, and nobody has the right to take that away from you.

Being the son of a southern Baptist minister, I used to watch and listen to how my father dealt with people and their families who were dealing with fatal illnesses. Something rubbed off. It's been very beneficial to me in preparing myself for my own death. It amazes me that our society feels that if they kill a sick animal they are being humane, but when a human is in horrible pain and very sick and makes that same choice, society says that it's immoral and against the law and against the Bible. We treat animals better in this society than we do humans.

What would I say to others?

I think what gets me through this illness is that, being a doctor, I'm very optimistic that right around the corner—right around the corner being two to three years—new drugs will be available that will prolong life and the quality of life for people with AIDS. I think that it will be much like people who have hepatitis B—they will be living with a chronic, treatable illness and live for 20 years in reasonably good health. I feel that the drugs we have now—AZT, DDI, and DDC—are attacking the virus in one area, and the new drugs will attack it in another area, so that it slows down the progression long enough for people to live for 10 to 20 years with the HIV virus. I don't think a drug will be available to kill the virus in the next few years, but I do feel that the disease will become a treatable, livable chronic disease. And on my optimistic days I want to be around for those drugs, so that I can live longer. So I fight for that day around the corner. I also have pessimistic days as well, and on those days I feel that I'm not going to be here. But everybody has and is entitled to good and bad days, and I am going to fight to be around for those new drugs.

The reason I'm willing to tell you anything about me is it's hard to do anything to me. It makes a great difference to be at a point in your life when you're *free.*

—*DR. DON HAGAN*

☐ Dr. Don Hagan died of AIDS on March 7, 1992, a few months after he expressed the words above. His childhood ambition was to be—a doctor.

□   □

> *"How could he possibly think that his opinion on homosexuality had anything to do with a devastating disease that was ravaging people, reducing them to skeletons and killing them?"*
>
> *—BRAD DAVIS ON RONALD REAGAN*
> for virtually ignoring AIDS during his administration

Actor Brad Davis found out that he was HIV-positive in 1985. At that time, Brad and his wife, Susan Bluestein, whom he had been with for 20 years, decided to keep his status a secret.

They kept their secret for six years, until Brad's death on September 8, 1991. One month after her husband's death, Susan agreed to be interviewed for this book to answer the inevitable question: *Why?*

Brad looked at the experience of Rock Hudson. There was also a rumor going around at one point that Burt Reynolds had AIDS, which was not true. Brad saw the experience that Burt Reynolds had gone through. He had not been able to get a job. There were hints in the industry that if an actor disclosed that he was HIV-positive, he might not be able to get a job. Don't forget what Brad had already gone through. He had had a very difficult time getting a job after he became sober because he had a reputation for drinking and drug abuse. He knew what it was like. He had had to prove to people all over again that he was sober and was going to be fine on the set. So he was not about to take a chance that he would have to suffer through that again. We had no way of knowing whether Hollywood would or wouldn't be supportive. And he just couldn't take that chance.

Brad had gone to Rome to do a movie. Before he left, he had given blood. I got *the* letter. I was stunned. I called him right away in Rome. He thought it was referring to somebody else. Unfortunately, he had to stay there to finish the show before we could do anything about it. When he got back, he was retested.

He did not get any medical treatment whatsoever until 1989. He was afraid of bringing anybody else into the circle. Anybody at all. It was hard to convince him that he could be treated anonymously. Finally, with enough encouragement from me—and his therapist—he did finally open himself a little to ask for help.

I think you have to understand that when Brad first found out, he was in exceptionally good health. He felt great. He looked great. He didn't know much about the disease. His information base—what could happen, how things developed—was not that strong at that time. A lot of the information people have today, they didn't have then. It was even before AZT. In the beginning, the information given to Brad was that he was a carrier, but since he was in such good health, he probably would never develop the disease. That's what the doctors thought at that time. As things progressed, I suppose, he wanted to believe that. We both did. Also, he still felt very good. He took very good care of himself, and I suppose for a while he believed that it was maybe true. Unfortunately, I have to say there was a certain amount of denial on both of our parts. I think that he felt that in some way he was fighting it off.

I believe he should have gotten treatment earlier. I wish he'd gotten treatment earlier. Once he went for treatment, he realized himself that he probably should have gone earlier. The drugs that are available might have saved him had he gone when he had more T-cells.

In 1989 he didn't have any symptoms, but he was starting to feel fatigued. Again, he put off getting treatment for as long as he could. Finally, he went on AZT. He stayed on that for a while, but he became a bit anemic. He was on Bactrim and later DDC.

In June 1991, after he came back from shooting his last movie, *A Habitation of Dragons,* Brad said that he would finally go public. I think he always had the idea that he would eventually go public. He felt that he owed it to other people out there who were suffering and to people who weren't yet. He started to write his book. You know, he was probably infected in 1979 and had survived for a long time. He felt that every year he lived was one more year that he could be around to show people you could live with this disease; every job he did would give people courage that you could live with this disease.

We still had hopes that he would rally.

And then he got a microbacteria, an opportunistic infection called MAI. It was the first serious opportunistic infection he had.

Most of Brad's friends never knew until the very, very end. Even at the end he didn't tell very many people. He told his best friend on July 4. There were a few who found out just shortly before he died and a couple he called from the hospital, but he really didn't tell people. I think he always knew that if his close friends knew, they'd be supportive, but he didn't want to have to put anybody in the position of having to keep the secret. What he didn't realize

118

was that his friends loved him and wanted to be there for him and could have been a great help and a great relief to him in a lot of ways.

We told our daughter, Alexandra, only a few days before he died. She had heard about AIDS. She just couldn't believe that it was that serious, that he was going to die. She thought that he would somehow get better. It was very, very hard. She was very upset. He was very upset. He was in terrible pain. It was a very hard day for all of us.

Every day, every hour, every moment that Brad was here with Alexandra and me I considered precious, because I knew that I was going to be left with a little girl who had been very close to her father. I was working very hard to make money to support us at that point. Things were very tough, so I was under a lot of stress myself. But I knew that I would eventually have this little girl who would be without a father, so I worked very hard to keep a positive attitude.

Over the years, I have to say, I really gained a lot of spiritual strength from Brad. Brad had really made peace with the situation. It had been a long haul for him. He had faced it, and then I was able to face it. I faced the fact that this was something I couldn't change, that the future was coming upon me.

What would I say to others?

For me, finally coming forth and telling the truth was a great relief. I feel very free. I feel a tremendous burden has been lifted. Hiding was very, very stressful, even though I agreed to do it at the time. It's a very freeing experience being able to finally tell the truth. I also really feel that it's absolutely urgent that people start to open up to these issues and talk about the reality that people are HIV-infected. So many people are hiding and so many people are afraid, and I'm not saying that they don't have good reason for that—they do—but as people start to come forward and tell the truth, this country will not be able to run and hide anymore. It is very difficult to live without being able to be free about your status. People have to be treated. People have to be allowed to work and live in a fair manner.

—*SUSAN BLUESTEIN*

☐ Brad Davis attained stardom with his acclaimed performance in the 1978 picture *Midnight Express.*
He died at the age of 41.

As of this writing, Susan Bluestein is writing a book to tell her story, the story of her husband, and the story of their secret life living with her husband's AIDS.

I had been ill with MAI last year, and I was out of work for about six weeks. I told my principal that I had AIDS. The school board knew, and a lot of the teachers knew. They were very supportive. When I decided to come back to work, I was going to work three days a week. I decided to go public so that I could hopefully educate parents and their children about AIDS. I wanted them to realize that it's not a death sentence and that people can live quite a while with the medications; that it is becoming more treatable. I also wanted to teach them that you can't get it just by being around someone without having sexual contact.

So I wrote a statement. I wanted to send a letter to the incoming kindergarten parents telling them that I had AIDS and that we would have a meeting, with health officials there to answer questions.

The following Tuesday, when we had the meeting scheduled, all the major networks were there. Our original intention was to have a small meeting with the parents where I would read my statement to them. When the press found out, there wasn't anything we could do to stop them, because we're government employees and it's a public meeting. We certainly didn't encourage the press

121

to be there. When I got there, there were all these TV cameras. I had thought maybe 50 parents would show up. There were about 300 of them. A lot of the parents whose kids I had the previous year showed up to support me. So did a lot of teachers. We had a panel on the stage in the auditorium, and I just sat down in the front row with some of the parents. My principal gave a brief opening statement, and then she introduced me. I got a standing ovation from all the parents who knew me. It was a real warm reception. I read my statement and sat down. Then they took questions from the audience. The first few were from parents who had previously had children in my class. They basically stood up and said that I was a good teacher and that they felt there was no reason that I shouldn't be teaching. Then more questions came up with concern from parents who thought that I should not be in the classroom. They weren't concerned that their children would get AIDS, but they were concerned that if I became ill or died it would be hard for the children to deal with emotionally.

I have 22 kids in my class. I think maybe four parents requested that their kids not be in my class.

What would I say to others?

I think having emotional support is very crucial. I am fortunate because I have my family supporting me. I also go to support groups and things of that nature. I certainly recommend to anyone who lives in a community that offers support groups to take advantage of them. If they don't have family support, at least seek out counseling of some kind. Letting out all of the emotional stress is very important. The first year I was diagnosed, I was working and taking care of my lover, who was ill. When he died, I was not yet public. I was not able to share that with my coworkers, and so I had to go through that trip alone. That certainly took its toll.

After my lover, David, died, I was not looking to get into a relationship. Then I met someone new, and I was actually pushing him off, especially when I found out that he was HIV-negative. But we fell in love. Before I moved in with him, I made him go through counseling with me. I wanted to make sure that he knew what the possibilities were. We've been together about two and a half years.

Coming out for me has been a very positive experience. I say, let as many people as you are comfortable with know. Every time I let someone know, it's a relief. Now everyone I know knows.

And it's important to have something to look forward to. I have an extremely busy occupation, and there's just so much that needs to be done. I think that kind of keeps me going. Fortunately, I love my job. I love working with the kids, and I get a lot of joy doing that. Kids can be very grounding. I also hope that I am making a difference to the kids. It's kind of scary how much influence you have with that age group. You know, everybody remembers their kindergarten teacher. But I certainly don't try to do anything to try to shape them. I try to encourage them to have open minds and to not judge people by anything other than how they are treated by them.

—TONY MARKS

☐ Tony Marks is 38 years old. As of this writing, his T-cell count is, in his own words, "10 . . . but [it's] been zero."

His childhood ambition was to be a guitar player, but he was born to be a teacher. Today he is still learning to live with AIDS and teaching lessons not found in textbooks.

One of the primary ways the AIDS virus is transmitted is from mother to child. Many of these children are later abandoned or orphaned. What happens to them? Where do they go? Who takes care of them?

People like Loretta and Thomas Lick do. In addition to their five children and seven grandchildren, the Licks have a family of foster children with AIDS. They recently adopted two of the children, a brother and sister named Tommy and Ashley.

Loretta, 46, and Thomas, 55, have lost about 10 of their foster children to AIDS.

My husband is a retired lithographic-ink chemist, and now he works for a refrigeration company. Now I primarily just stay home and take care of the kids. It's a 24-hour-a-day job.

It's hard to say how many children with AIDS we've fostered, because over the years they really wouldn't say a child had AIDS. When the kids would die, it would be from "pneumonia" or some other complication. They really wouldn't say AIDS. Even nowadays they won't say it. The doctors like to use the term *immune deficiency*, because they're more comfortable with it. These children are still called "drug babies" or "medically fragile." When a case-worker calls you up, he says, "We have a drug child."

I've been a foster parent for 27 years. We've had over 300 children in our home. We started with the infectious-disease children about eight years ago because nobody else would take them. We started with a child who had syphilis, and our house just kind of became known as the infectious home. Great title, huh?

When we got our Ashley, she was five months old. Ashley Anne. We were told that she was a "preemie," a cocaine, heroin, fetal-alcohol baby. Her mother had abandoned her in the emergency room. They didn't tell us that she was an AIDS baby. You just don't know. You take these drug children into your home, but you know that all drug children are primary candidates for AIDS. You do it with fear. You say, "I hope to God this isn't an AIDS child." A lot of the foster parents who find out that the child has AIDS will call up the caseworker and say, "Find somebody else."

We adopted Ashley and her brother because they wanted to put them in an institution. And this was the only way to save them. When the children get really bad, the state would rather put them in an institution.

I take the terminally ill and the HIV and AIDS children. I do not know why. I just have an affinity for them. I take them because nobody wants them. They're kind of outcasts. Right now, we're an outcast family. We're outcasts in the straight community. We're accepted into the gay community. We go to church in the gay and lesbian community. We do everything there, because the straight community does not accept us.

We've lost a lot of friends. Our neighbors refuse to let their children play with our children. Our kids aren't allowed in certain schools. Our son, who's HIV-positive, cannot go to day care. His name is Thomas. He's three and a half years old.

125

Our daughter Ashley isn't supposed to be here. They told us she wouldn't live to see her first birthday. She's now hit four and a half years. But we know that we don't have a long time with her. I recently signed a "Do Not Resuscitate" on her, which is very hard to do, because you know that the end is coming. But you have to do it. We've brought her back with CPR nine times, but the virus has infected every organ in her body. You know, her eyesight is gone, her hearing is gone, she's got lymph nodes under her arms the size of golf balls, she's in a lot of pain. And when we go to the clinic the doctors see her for maybe a couple of minutes—but you live it 24 hours a day.

She's constantly sick with simple little things like an ear infection that can turn into pneumonia. Sinus infections. Eye infections. Even from cutting her fingernails she can get an infection. Her skin is *so* delicate. And she bleeds.

My mother will not talk to me. She will not touch my children. When she first saw my children she went, "Oh, they're black." Our daughter is black, white, and Asian. Her brother is black, white, and Hispanic. I haven't seen a white child in years.

We've gotten mixed feelings from our natural children. One of the girls says, "Mom, you're doing a great thing." The other one tends to ignore the whole situation like they didn't exist. Our daughter in Arizona does not know what kind of children we take. Our oldest son is in the service; he doesn't care. And our other son is gay and very supportive. It bothers me because some of my grandchildren I won't be able to see. But my children know that I'm there for them and these children need me *now*. My natural children have had me for years and years, but these little guys don't have me for long.

People ask me how I have the strength to do this.

If you've ever held a sick child, a really sick child, like our

Ashley Anne, you can have the rottenest day in the world where everything goes wrong. I might be up with her for 36 hours straight because she's in so much pain, and I have to keep turning her and stripping her bed, the whole thing; and she'll just kind of have this look on her face, this peaceful look. And I pick her up and things are all right again. She kind of gives me the strength to go on. We call them peace babies. I've sat on panels with parents who've had older children die from AIDS. And they said when things got really bad, their children seemed to give off this aura of peace, as if they were saying, "See, Mom, it's all right. Here's my strength to go on another day."

You get a lot less sleep. Moneywise, we're always, really, just going, because a lot of things are not covered. When Ashley is sick there are experimental drugs they have to put her on that are not covered by CCS [California Children's Services] or Medi-Cal or anything. So without support groups like Tuesday's Child helping us, we would really be devastated. Sometimes we are really devastated, and my husband says, "OK, you have to go out and find some extra work," or, "We'll just have to pull in. We don't pay this, we don't pay that." But it gives us the strength to cope with other things. You become more spiritual, you know? You believe in miracles.

Ashley understands what's going on, even though the virus has totally destroyed her brain. We don't hide it from the children. Tommy knows that his sister is very sick. In fact, a couple of weeks ago, he was watching the commercial on television for Baby Alive. It was a battery-operated doll that does everything. After watching it, Tommy was trying to get his sister to sit up like Baby Alive. I said, "Tommy, what are you doing?" He said, 'I'm putting batteries into Ashley to make her better."

What would I say to other parents who are considering adopting or fostering children with the virus?

Well, you've got to have a lot of stamina. You've got to have a lot of time. And you've got to be willing to fight the system. When your child is labeled "no potential" or "terminal," the system doesn't want to give you anything. They say, "Well, why should we waste money on this? Why should we give you money for a wheelchair when the child only has six months to live?" Or, "Why should we give you this medication when it could go to another child?"

And it takes something special to know that when you take these children, they're not going to live. When people adopt children they adopt them for a lifetime. They're planning weddings and grandchildren and everything. These children are not going to have that. These children are not going to have weddings.

—LORETTA LICK

☐ Loretta and Thomas Lick are still fighting the heartache and bigotry inherent in fostering children with the virus. Nevertheless, as of this writing, they were planning to open their home to three more children with AIDS.

Two recent events dramatically altered the course of 33-year-old Joel Rothschild's life. First, in 1989, he tested HIV-positive. Then, in October 1991, he and his lover, Kevin, were badly beaten in an alleged assault by an enraged cab driver.

During the beating and its aftermath, Joel's blood intermingled with Kevin's. At the time, Kevin was HIV-negative.

I always knew that I was different. I figured out I was gay when I was 13. I knew that I had to do something different, that I had to be independent. So I started going to school around the clock. I went to prep school, and I used to go to school during summers to get ahead. I graduated from high school at 16 and was out of college by the time I was 19. I was obsessed with getting out of school. High school was so straight. I wanted to move to the big city.

I started with a Porsche 944 in my early 20s. Then I went to a Jaguar and then to a Mercedes and then to a Rolls-Royce. I always thought I'd have my first hundred thousand dollars in the bank and I'd be rich, followed by my second hundred thousand and then my third hundred thousand. I thought more money would make me happy.

Then, all of a sudden, the day I tested positive, I realized that I might not have the time to get to the million dollars I thought would make me happy. And so I just let go of it all. I said to myself, Thank the universe that I have worked this hard. I'm comfortable. I don't have to worry about losing my job. I don't have to worry about paying the rent, because the condo is paid for. I let go of the obsession. And I let go of needing *things* to be happy. Life became a lot simpler, and things became a lot less important.

Now I do volunteer work for a lot of AIDS charities, and I do political action work with ACT-UP and the National Gay and Lesbian Task Force.

Actually, I've been an activist since I was 15. When I was younger, I didn't realize how prejudiced the world was. I did protesting and marching and charity work, and I worked on the Dade County ordinance that Anita Bryant worked against. At 15, I marched with Leonard Matlovich [the U.S. Air Force sergeant who came out of the closet and appeared on the cover of *Time* magazine], and a lot of people told me how special it was that I was out of the closet at 15.

Before I opened my own business, I was fired from a job because I was gay. My boss accused me of being gay, and I told him I was. I was so naive in accepting myself.

Since I tested HIV-positive, I've worked harder [for gay rights] because I realize that I may have less time. And if I'm going to die from this disease, I want to leave the world a little bit better for other people and for younger gay people. Because, boy, when I was a teenager, I was a teenager alone.

I'm still a fairly young person at 33, but I've been out of the closet for a long time. And when you look back on it, not a lot has changed for gay people. God, there's still so much hostility, so much hatred, and there's pandemic violence against gay people.

It happened on October 1, 1991. I was marching with my lover, Kevin, in the AB-101 protest. [AB-101 was a gay-rights bill that had been approved by the California legislature but was then vetoed by Gov. Pete Wilson after he had initially vowed to support it. Wilson's veto launched a nightly series of protests in the state and galvanized the gay community at large.] We decided to film the protest for a documentary that we were making.

Everything was fine. The protest was peaceful, spiritual. But there was a cab whose driver was trying to push his way through a gridlock of people, and this cab hit Kevin in the leg. It was kind of scary, but Kevin stood up and everything seemed OK. He tried to catch the cab driver's face on-camera, so he turned the camera on, which had a light on it, and the guy came out of his car with a leaded flashlight, a "mag light." It's like a leaded pipe. He hit Kevin across the side of the face, and he hit the camera and shattered a part of it. Then he hit Kevin on the other side of the face, and Kevin stumbled and started bleeding.

It's really hard to see someone you love get hurt. I freaked for two seconds. I was about 10 feet away. Then I ran to Kevin and the guy hit me behind my head with the pipe. I went unconscious, and the guy continued to beat me.

I remember waking up with a crowd of people around me, putting pressure on my head. Blood was pouring out. The pain was unbelievable. I had to have 50 to 60 stitches in my head. My ribs were bruised. I had welts all over my body. Kevin needed stitches on his face and had cuts all over his arms.

The police weren't even going to arrest the cab driver, but the crowd surrounded him and forced the police to arrest him. We're prosecuting him under the fullest extent of the law. Because we're gay, because we're out of the closet, we've had problems with the district attorney not wanting to prosecute him. But there were 35 eyewitnesses. We're standing up against gay-bashing, because we've learned what it's like to be a victim for the first time.

And what have I learned? I've learned how to enjoy life. I really like classical music. I listen all the time, and I'm able to enjoy it now more than ever before. I never knew how to relax before. I used to worry about my looks, and now I just don't worry about them anymore.

What would I tell other people who are HIV-positive?

Not to trust your doctor. Also, no drugs. No drinking. No smoking. And live a stress-free life. Arrange your life to give you the time to rest. Even if you have to live a little bit less. You have to respect your body.

Read *everything*. Call 1-800-TRIALS-A and get the *AMFAR AIDS/ HIV Treatment Directory* that comes out quarterly and read it cover to cover. Subscribe to the *AIDS Treatment News*. Subscribe to the *Persons With AIDS Treatment News* out of New York. You have to read and read and read and read and read. You have to learn how this virus works. There are so many charlatans out there, it's really disgusting.

I think it's important not to lie to anyone. Lying is making excuses. There's no need for it. You have to be honest with yourself first, and then you have to be honest with the people around you, because the best part of the experience of life is being able to come together with a person and understand what they're going through. One thing I've learned with this virus is to develop empathy and compassion. If you live your life without empathy, you're not really living at all. Well, you've living, but you're living in a prison.

And what a waste of life that is.

—JOEL ROTHSCHILD

☐ Joel Rothschild is still fighting the good fight. His lover, Kevin, is still testing HIV-negative.

I was pregnant at the time and felt that I needed to be tested. In 1989, when I was about six months pregnant, they called me on the phone and told me that I was HIV-infected.

It was a drastic change in my life, the worst nightmare you could possibly imagine. They started me on 1,200 milligrams of AZT a day. They had no regard for my health, they were just concerned about the virus being passed to the child. Consequently, they almost killed me in the process. Now I only do vitamin therapy. My T-cells have increased since I stopped the AZT. You have to have a very close watch over your own health.

As for the baby's father, we weren't going together. It was a one-night stand. I'm a lesbian.

I had a lot of bad things happen to me in the process of being diagnosed and getting access to health care. Simple things, like trying to find someone to deliver the baby, were hard. We ran up against a lot of brick walls, a lot of discrimination, and a lot of judgmental people.

So I turned to activism. I've gotten real political, and I know that AIDS is very political. I'm very open about my status. I'm very open about my past history and my present. It seems to help me, being honest with myself and with others. It seems to make me stronger. Activism is a way for me to channel my anger, plus contribute to society and educate people and bring their awareness up. I figured if I ran up against that many walls, that much hardship, I couldn't imagine other women going through what I was going through. Some women aren't as strong as I am.

What would I say to other women?

It definitely changes your life. But it's up to you to empower yourself. Just how much change are you going to allow this virus to do to you? The main thing is, what comforts me the most, is educating myself. That's what gives me, really, a lot of strength. I'm very well educated on the issue now. Before I wasn't. When I was diagnosed, I knew nothing about HIV. It always helps if you know what's happening.

If I can save one person from being infected, it makes my life all worth it.

I've been in a relationship with a woman now for two years. We're extremely cautious. We practice safer sex. We're both real educated on the issue, so we're not putting her at risk at all. We don't exchange body fluids. Simple as that.

You know, lesbians do drugs. Lesbians do sleep with men. I knew I was at risk. I just didn't think it would happen to me.

—MARY LUCEY

☐ Mary Lucey is 33 years old. As of this writing, she is still healthy and is working full-time as an AIDS activist.

Her daughter, born two years ago, is HIV-negative.

I never thought it was going to happen to me. You know, it always happens to others, but not to us. So when it happened, it was a big shock. And I had already seen a lot of my friends die. Some of them died very peacefully, but some died in a very troubled way, after five years of constant deterioration. I felt that when the time came for me, I would commit suicide and prevent the deterioration.

But my second thought was, in the meantime, I'm not going to sit under a tree and wait to die. I have responsibilities to the life and breath that I do have. I will try to live my life with as much quality as I can. Then, as things progressed, the thought of suicide was consciously eliminated, little by little.

We are taught as human beings the victimization philosophy— the "poor little me" philosophy. But I stopped saying, "Why me?" and I started to say, "What could be the lesson hidden in this?" I took full responsibility for what was happening in my life. I believe that what is going on in our physical bodies is just mirroring what is going on in our consciousness. And before any physical healing can take place, the healing of the spirit must be considered first. I found great empowerment in that.

One of the first things I did after my diagnosis was to work with a nutritionist. My food intake has been very conscious in the last 10 or 12 years, on the very healthy side, but I wanted to make it even more so. So I started working with this lady who changed my diet, primarily to cure the candida that I had. I had had skin problems prior to my diagnosis for which the dermatologist gave me antibiotics. But of course the antibiotics were the main thing that caused the candida, so it was a catch-22. The nutritionist said that I'd have to stop the antibiotics; the doctor said that I'd have to take the antibiotics for the rest of my life. But when I stopped the AZT, I also stopped the antibiotics. And with the proper diet, all the candida disappeared. All the skin problems that I had had also disappeared. I had been wearing turtleneck shirts in the middle of August.

What would I say to other people with AIDS?

I believe that this illness has a tendency to absorb our lives, and we *become* AIDS. We forget our own identity and become AIDS. I think that we should keep our life going with all of the other stuff that creates who we are. I know it's difficult at times.

One of my needs used to be to have this incredibly romantic and idealized relationship with another man. That has never happened. I have had wonderful, idealized relationships with women, but I haven't have them with men. After I was diagnosed and until very recently, my sorrow was that I wouldn't have time to accomplish that. And then, all of a sudden, in recent months, that need has subsided. I guess, as my relationship with myself is getting better, that need is being eliminated. Today, if it happens, great. It'll be wonderful. But if it doesn't happen, I'm still whole and wonderful myself.

I remember, about 15 or 20 years ago, when I was going through dramatic periods of my life, I had friends who used to tell me, "You must love yourself more." And my jaw would drop and I would say, "My God! I think I'm one of the most selfish people in the world!" I've learned that loving oneself has nothing to do with selfishness.

Today, when I happen to pass a mirror, I stop and tell myself how much I love myself. In the beginning, that may have been an exercise, but now it's very genuine. It comes from the gut.

—PANOS CHRISTI

☐ Panos Christi, 54, was an actor, director, and poet originally from Greece. He was diagnosed with Kaposi's sarcoma and AIDS in April 1988. He passed away on April 25, 1992.

❏   ❏

I tested HIV-positive in August of 1990. Since then I've been fighting a constant battle between wanting to keep a sense of normalcy in my life, in terms of making future plans and having career goals and things like that, versus—how can I say it?—just sort of letting things go and living for the present. I don't mean that in a decadent way. I guess maybe living a little more just for pleasure, just for enjoying the pleasures of the moment, rather than worrying about what's coming down the line in terms of future plans and goals, as most people my age do.

I'm in nursing school now, and I found out I was positive about two weeks before I was supposed to have started school. I had to do a lot of soul-searching at that point to decide whether—if I have a limited amount of time left to spend on this planet—I really want to spend the next two or three years of my life working myself to the bone, working toward a long-term career goal. I pretty much decided that in order to have a sense of purpose and have any kind of desire to continue on with life, you have to have these goals. You have to have a reason for getting up in the morning, and my reason for getting up in the morning is, you know, becoming a nurse. I'm currently working in the special-care unit at Century City Hospital.

And yeah, I could've gone on as a nurse's assistant, my current role, and just sort of cruised on that, but it isn't enough. You need to keep moving forward in spite of the sword of doom hanging over your head all the time.

I had started out as a volunteer at AIDS Project Los Angeles. At the time, I was in a totally different career field, working in publicity in the entertainment business. I was not enraptured with my career and what I was doing, and all around me my friends were getting sick and dying.

I was thinking, This is ridiculous. I've got to do something about this. I can't just sit here and pretend it's not happening. So I got involved with APLA and worked on the hotline for a while and then decided I wanted more direct contact with people with AIDS. My strengths, I feel, really lie more in personal kinds of interactions with people, and I thought, Well, what can I do in connection with this organization where I can really get close to people? They had a hospital-visitation program, which I got involved with. I went through all of their training and whatnot and was assigned to Century City Hospital as a volunteer. I got so involved in it I was spending an awful lot of time there, probably between 10 and 15 hours a week. In addition to really enjoying being with the patients and acting in my capacity as a volunteer, I got real interested in medicine, and the staff there sensed my interest and began to allow me to participate in things in a greater capacity. Eventually, as the unit grew and expanded, there was a need for having nurses' assistants and ward clerks on the floor. Prior to that, there hadn't been enough patients to justify that extra personnel. They essentially created a position for me and another volunteer, who was as involved and committed as I was to the unit.

It's funny. When you start nursing school, they ask you what you might think your long-term goals are in terms of specialty. There

139

has never been any question in my mind that HIV nursing, AIDS nursing, is the direction that I have to go. It's what I've committed my life to.

I go to school every day, Monday through Friday. I have classes on Monday and Wednesday; Tuesday I spend studying in a nurse's laboratory; Thursday and Friday I'm studying in a hospital. And I work at Century City Hospital on the weekends—two 12-hour shifts. It's every day, all day.

How has working as a nurse's assistant helped me get through my own diagnosis?

I'm not quite sure how I could have coped without this [nursing] experience. Some people might think it's scary to constantly be bombarded with the realities of the disease. On the other hand, I'm comforted by it. At least I feel I'm in possession of all the information that's currently known about it, and that gives me a sense of power over the disease that I might not otherwise have.

What would I say to others?

You've got to get involved. You've got to do something, anything. If the way you want to get involved is to go out and protest, you know, the repeal of gay-rights legislation or the lack of AIDS funding, if that's your way of coping with this, fine, do that. Get involved with a volunteer organization. Get involved with food organizations like Project Angel Food. If that's your bag, if you want to deliver meals to people with AIDS, whatever, just do something.

The patients I've seen who have the most trouble coping with their diagnosis of full-blown AIDS are people who have more or less stuck their head in the sand and just kind of ignored it as an issue in their life. They're the people who don't deal with it. The people who get out there and fight, who stay involved and stay active and learn as much as they can, are the ones who have more satisfying lives in terms of whatever time they have left. They lead full, rich, complete, satisfying lives, and when it's time for them to make their exit, the exit isn't as frightening.

There was always a part of me that was torn. Based on my upbringing, I always thought that success was something you could count, like money or power or fame. There was a part of me very early on that was seeking those kinds of gratifications in life. What I've come to learn through all this mess that we're in right now is that that's not where it's at at all. The true gratification in life comes from being with people, helping other people. It's the best kind of high there is.

Don't bury your head in the sand. AIDS is going to touch everybody, straight and gay, every walk of life, every part of the country, every part of the world. You've got to get involved, and you've got to do something.

What would I say to other health-care professionals who refuse to treat people with AIDS?

I don't understand how anyone could enter this profession and not be willing to treat people who are sick. I mean, in my heart, what I would say to them, I guess, is, "I think you should leave. I think this is not something you should be doing, because you are missing the fundamental essence of what it is to care for another human being."

What would I say to other health-care professionals who do treat people with AIDS?

The first thing I would say to them is that the need for the care they provide is only going to increase, and we're going to need more and more people who are willing to do the kind of work that they do. So it's vital that they take care of themselves physically, emotionally, spiritually.

I always feel privileged and honored to be allowed into a patient's room. It's like I'm being invited to do something very intimate with them. I've always felt honored that they would allow me and respect me enough to allow me to do that, to touch them, to do the things that I need to do to make them more comfortable. It's a fantastic feeling to be so trusted by another human being.

And I would say to them that when you leave work every day, you really have the sense that you've made a difference in people's lives.

—*SCOTT BIGGAM*

☐ Scott Biggam, who can teach even the most esteemed doctor a thing or two about health care, is 36 years old. As of this writing he is still healthy, still working as a nurse's assistant, and making a difference.

A year before I found out, somebody I had been seeing at work for about a year came up to me and told me that he had gotten a letter saying that he was HIV-positive. When he told me, I walked away from him. It wasn't very nice, I know, but I didn't believe him. I didn't want to believe him.

I was with an HMO [health maintenance organization] and went to a general practitioner who took some blood tests. Then my gynecologist said to me, "Your doctor has a feeling that you may be HIV-positive." I just couldn't accept that. They wanted me to take the test, and I didn't want to. I didn't want to know.

At work I had a high-pressure job. I had a lot of people working under me, a lot of responsibility. And I was trying to get a job done. But it got so bad that some days I couldn't drive the car. I had to stop wearing heels because I had no equilibrium. In the ladies' room they had a lounge, and I'd have to lie down. And I'd black out. When I could drive the car, half the time I didn't even remember how I had driven to work. I couldn't even remember where I parked the car. And at my job I worked with numbers, and I was writing them backward. I was a mess. This went on for about a year.

I finally took the test, and the doctor told me, "You've been exposed to the AIDS virus." I walked out of there, and I had to go back to work. I was in shock.

I was living with somebody at the time. I was terrified. I couldn't tell him. How could I tell him, when I couldn't even tell myself?

Finally, about a month later, I told a friend of mine who said, "Well, do you have AIDS or are you just HIV-positive?" I said, "Well, I don't know." You know, it never occurred to me that there was even a difference. That's how much I knew. So he said, "Well, why don't you call your doctor and find out?" I got up the courage to finally call my doctor and say to him, "Am I HIV-positive or do I have AIDS?" And that's when he said to me, "Well, it's *suspect.*" That's what he said. So I went to see him and said, "Well, don't you think I should be taking something, or be doing something about this?" He said, "Oh, no, not until you get really sick." I found out later that my T-cells at that time were only 150.

It just didn't make any sense to me at all. I was not getting better. I never felt good. Always tired, night sweats, I'd wake up soaking wet, and I never had energy.

What did I do? I changed doctors.

By the time I got to another doctor, my T-cells had plunged to 75. This one told me, "Yes, you do have AIDS" and told me he was going to put me on AZT. With an HMO, there's so much red tape that it took about three months for me to get it.

I had just started on AZT when I came down with pneumocystis on New Year's Eve of 1989. I went to the emergency room, but they didn't know what to do with me. They took X rays, and the woman said to me, "I just don't understand why you want to know if you have pneumonia." I told her I had AIDS, and my friend yelled at her, "She says she has AIDS!" The woman looked, went, "Oh!" and ran out of the room and down the hall. She was so frantic. Finally, they told me they didn't think it was pneumonia and sent me back home. I had a fever of 104 that night and my friends had to keep my temperature down.

For three days I sat at home thinking that I didn't have pneumonia. Then I went in for a doctor's appointment and they took another X ray. He couldn't read it, so he had to have a specialist come in. They put me immediately into the hospital. I had pneumocystis. I was also anemic.

I became very resentful toward people, including my friends. I resented that they were healthy, and I didn't know how to deal with it. And I *love* men. I love going out, and I love having a good time. I've always been like that. I have not been able to have a permanent relationship, you know, but I still really like being with a man. I felt that this had been taken away from me. So I rebelled. And I felt that my friends didn't approve of things I was doing, that I still wanted to date. I even had an argument with one of my friends, and it became really ugly.

I would say to a guy to use a rubber. But he'd say, his comment would be, "Oh, no! Not with you. Why would I want to do that?" And I'd think to myself, They don't even want to help themselves. They hear about it all the time. They tell you on the radio. They tell you on the TV. Be careful, be careful, be careful. So why are they being so stupid? And I felt, I'm not out here to save them all. At first I felt I should. At first I felt like I needed to be really good and try to save the world. Then I thought, f—k it. These are the things that I went through. So I just did what I could. That was it. I felt that if it wasn't from me, maybe they'd get it from someone else.

I went through a lot of changes, a lot of emotional, mixed-up feelings. Now I've gotten to a better place. It took a long time.

Now I tell them that I'm positive. If they don't accept it, then they don't accept it. But I would rather be with somebody else who is positive, because otherwise, in my head, while we're having sex, I'm wondering, is he thinking about *it?* Is he scared? Is he this, is he that? And it ruins the whole thing. He may not be thinking that at all. But I am. So, you know, it doesn't work.

Just the other day, I could tell one of my neighbors was interested in me, you know? I turned to him and said, "You know, having sex nowadays is more than black and white. There's more to it. And anyway, I'm HIV-positive." I said it just like I was going to the corner for cigarettes or something. He didn't react badly at all—quite well, in fact. He changed his mind, though.

But there will be people who are still interested even though they're scared. I met somebody in the doctor's office, a girl who met somebody who's not HIV-positive. She is. They're getting married. You know, it's the luck of the draw. Some people are lucky.

I meet men through placing ads with AIDS Project Los Angeles. I tried it once through *Pennysaver,* and they called me up and said they would not take my ad unless I changed the wording of "HIV-positive." I said, "What do you suggest that I do? What is the wording you suggest I use?" And they said, "Well, compassionate, open-minded." I said, "No, never mind. I don't want to." I mean, I don't want lies any more. I can't live that way. I can't live with a lie. I don't want to see somebody for a couple of weeks or a month and then have to break the news. It stresses you out too much. I'd rather tell them right off or just not go out at all.

What would I say to others?

You have to fight. You have to believe. This is your life. You know when your doctor can be doing things better. There is an instinct. *You know.* You know if they're brushing you off. You know if they care or don't care. And when you feel you're not getting support from that medical person, you've got to get out of there and find somebody else. You have to. You've got to fight for your life because no one else is going to do it for you.

I think some of these doctors are scared shitless. As soon as my first doctor walked into the room, this veil came over his eyes. He just didn't want to know about AIDS. He was totally ignorant and didn't want to show his ignorance.

And, I would say, don't hide it. Because you might find that the person you're hiding it from might have it also. The person you're standing next to could have it. When they say, "If you want to see someone with AIDS, look in the mirror"—it's the truth.

—DIANNE RICE

☐ Dianne Rice is 47 years old. At the time of this writing she had been on DDI for 10 months. "Since I've been on DDI," says Dianne, "I've been—knock on wood—pretty damn healthy."

"**P**ositive" always meant something good when I was growing up. Now the word seems almost synonymous with despair. Why not another word for being infected with HIV? Maybe "subjected," you know, like being subjected to a bad perm. I walked into a bar in my hometown a few years ago and gave them "fetching Californian," tanned, bi-level, open-mouthed smiles. While there, I met a prospective—well, you know. So we exchanged pleasantries and phone numbers, and then he whispered in my ear, "I'm negative, so we can party." I laughed and he walked away. I wished I had said, "I only see men who are positive" (as in about themselves). I'm a subjected, or positive, or anything-else-they-come-up with person who has tried for a long time to stay clear of labeling. I'm not cruising up the river "De-Nile," just staying clear of the arrows.

The hardest part of living with HIV for me has been watching my friends go and taking mental notes of what I do and don't want. I think being a person with HIV allows me to experience the pain of others and learn how to avoid regret. Before I found out my results, I found myself in regret over my sexual overconduct, the way I treated my family, the things I had or had not said to old loves, et cetera. Watching my friends go, I have been privileged to be an onlooker as well as a caregiver. I am learning some fine-tuning on how to treasure what I have. I'm able to laugh at my own sometimes dramatic interpretations about how *life* is treating *me,* and now I'm able to think more of "How am *I* treating *life?*"

What would I say to others?

I've learned from my friends what I do and don't want to happen. One friend really lost his dignity in a big way with major dementia. I'd buy the book *Final Exit* and learn more before I slipped into that position. Another friend, Scott, on the other hand, kept his faculties until the end. The day before he died, he was cracking jokes. I've just really observed and learned and discovered through them. I really do try to stop and smell the roses. I really enjoy my friends. I enjoy my lover. I enjoy my kitten. I'm pampering myself and allowing myself to really enjoy what's around me. I know it sounds really yellow-brick-road, but I've watched some of my friends do it—and that's the way to go.

—*MIKE DONNICI*

☐ Mike Donnici is 21 years old. He was diagnosed HIV-positive in July 1990. Today he remains positive in the best sense of the word.

On June 10, 1989, 38-year-old Robert Enright died of AIDS. He left behind his two teenage sons, a group of close friends, and his mother, Ruth Sims.

I remember two Christmases ago, he came home and spent the holidays with my daughter and me. And both these Christmases he had some kind of bronchial disturbance. He'd get cold or flu symptoms. Even before that, he was in the hospital. I thought maybe he had pneumonia, but he said, no, that it was just a bad cold.

He always denied it to me right up to near the end.

From the way he denied it to me, he must not have discussed it much with the boys, either. I know that they knew he was sick, but I really think they were too absorbed in their own worlds.

Bobby was 10 years old when Bob and his wife got divorced. And I guess Walter must've been eight. They lived with their mother for a while. Then there was some kind of trouble at school, and there was a possibility that they would be put into a foster home. When Bob found out about this, he took the children and they lived with him for five years before he became ill.

They knew their father was gay. When he took them, he had a beautiful apartment for them to live in. And he put them in school. The boys were too young, I think, to understand very much [about their father's homosexuality]. And they were thriving in school. Bob had a long-term relationship [with another man] that was really significant, and at that point in time the four of them really thrived.

Bob was planning a big party for his birthday on May 24, 1989. He hired a cabaret, some musicians, and several vocalists. They rehearsed several times. On May 15, as he was walking home with his cane, he collapsed. He crawled through the alley to his home, and then he called me. He had lost control of his bowels and everything. I kind of got hysterical and said, "I'll call a doctor." He said he had just called his doctor and he couldn't be reached. Well, *I* called the doctor and finally got through to him to arrange for an ambulance. Meanwhile Bob also called his friend Jim, who lived closer. Jim helped clean Bob up and had him ready for when the ambulance got there. Then I rushed to the hospital, and when I got there Bob was still in the emergency room. Finally, when they got him settled in a room, they had to take him off the AZT immediately because he had become totally anemic. I said to the doctor, "Well, won't the infections start now?" And he said, "I can't leave him on AZT." And it all went downhill from there, because he was no longer on AZT.

Bob wouldn't cancel the party. The hospital threatened that his medical insurance wouldn't cover him if he left the hospital. Finally, some of his real-estate friends, very wealthy, said they would under-write that day in the hospital if the insurance company wouldn't pay. So my daughter went to his apartment and got his tuxedo and cummerbund. They picked him up in a limousine that had been ordered by one of my daughter's friends. We were all there. I got up on the stage and told everybody that he would be coming. And then he came in with his cane. He walked in and everybody got up. There were about 80 people there.

Bob had planned to walk into the room in drag and sing "Where the Boys Are." He had a whole list of songs that he was going to sing. But, you know, that didn't happen. He sat at a little round table, and little by little, two at a time, one at a time, people walked up to him and hugged and kissed him. For the final song, we all surrounded him and sang "That's What Friends Are For." We were holding hands and swaying, and everyone was crying.

The next morning I went to the hospital, and he was sitting there with his friend Sandy, watching the video of the party. He was crying and said, "Mom, this is the happiest time of my life."

What have I learned?

I've been around this topic [her son's homosexuality] since my son was 16. I don't know if I was any more understanding or accepting than anybody else. Maybe it was because I saw no alternative. Either you lose your child or you accept your child. So I didn't have a hard time accepting it. And I kind of think my children appreciated that. What I've learned is to accept your children, whatever they are or however they live. I've never been able to understand all the meanness in people. My son was very talented. My son was a beautiful soul. He was kind, and everyone loved him.

I have learned more about AIDS.

Before Bob died, I didn't even know what *pneumocystis* meant.

—RUTH SIMS

I knew when I went to take the AIDS test that I had it. I had been sick off and on for a while, and when I finally went to the doctor, the test results came back saying that I was positive and that I had only 47 T-cells. The first thing I thought of were my sons. I have two sons from an early marriage.

About a month after I received my test results, I came down with pneumocystis. Once I was over that, I started aerosolized pentamidine, but a week later I got pneumocystis for the second time. Then I started Bactrim and have been on that for almost a year and a half. It has worked very well for me. Currently, I'm also on AZT. I have lived with zero to seven T-cells for the past 18 months, but I really have had no problems. When I was diagnosed with full-blown AIDS, I quit my job because of stress. I've lost about 60 pounds. I look ill, but I feel great.

It was on November 22, 1988, the day before my 43rd birthday, that I was told I was going on a journey, one that I may not return from. On this journey I would meet an array of people from all walks of life, some good, some bad, and some who just didn't give a damn, as in all journeys. And so I went not knowing what to expect or how long it would take, and thus started my journey with

AIDS. My first trip on this journey was to go home and tell my loved ones—mother, brothers, sisters, friends—not knowing what the outcome would be. And thus started the disbelief, sorrow, pity, confusion, and pain that went with this trip.

What would I say to others?

Simple: Don't give up and don't give in! I was told by the doctors after my second diagnosis of pneumocystis that I had one to six months left to live. That was two years ago. Today I keep very active. I take a strong multivitamin and have a hell of a strong, positive attitude. Don't buy into the disease. Once you are diagnosed, don't sit around and think about when you will get this illness or that illness, because you will get it. That's what I did. Once I was diagnosed as positive I kept thinking, actually waiting to get pneumocystis. I got it within a month. Be careful of what you wish for or think about because you will get it. I won't allow myself to be around negative people, be it family, friends, or doctors. I listen to a lot of stress tapes, and I talk to God every day. Don't listen to people who tell you you can't do this or that. I was told not to cut grass, but I cut grass seven hours a day, twice a week.

I have also tried to educate the people in my area. I have written articles for the local newspapers about AIDS and people with AIDS, and I know it's made a difference.

My current project is to get Michael Bolton's song "When I'm Back on My Feet Again" as the national anthem for people with AIDS. This song gave me the strength, courage, and inspiration to fight and go on. And I know that it has done the same for other people with AIDS as well. So I wrote to Michael Bolton's fan club to ask him if I could get the rights to the song. Michael passed the letter on to the writer and owner of the song, Diane Warren, who gave me the permission. I have letters from her and her attorney giving me permission to use the song, so I sent copies of their letters, along with my own, to President Bush asking if he could give his approval for this to back it up in some way—and he's never responded. That song says it all for me, and I know that it does for other people. So I listen to Michael's song and it gives me the energy and the inspiration to go on living . . . trying . . . and fighting. I won't give up trying to get this song approved and heard and known as the national song for people with AIDS.

—JOSEPH NOTO

□ The lyrics that have been so meaningful in the life of Joseph Noto are reprinted below.

When I'm Back on My Feet Again
By Diane Warren

Gonna break these chains around me
Gonna learn to fly again
May be hard, may be hard
But I'll do it
When I'm back on my feet again

Soon these tears will all be dryin'
Soon these eyes will see the sun
Might take time, might take time
But I'll see it
When I'm back on my feet again

155

When I'm back on my feet again
I'll walk proud down this street again
And they'll all look at me again
And they'll see that I'm strong

Gonna hear the children laughing
Gonna hear the voices sing
Won't be long, won't be long
Till I hear them
When I'm back on my feet again

Gonna feel the sweet light of heaven
Shining down its light on me
One sweet day, one sweet day
I will feel it
When I'm back on my feet again

And I'm not gonna crawl again
I will learn to stand tall again
No I'm not gonna fall again
'Cause I'll learn to be strong

Soon these tears will all be dryin'
Soon these eyes will see the sun
Won't be long, won't be long
Till I see it
When I'm back on my feet again
When I'm back on my feet again
I'll be back on my feet again

At a time when former child stars are receiving exposure for their dubious exploits, it is significant to note the growth of Alison Arngrim. Little Nellie Olson is not so little anymore.

I'm stoned on Sudafed, so I can't be responsible for everything I say.

As many of you know, if you recognized the name Arngrim—who the hell has a name like that?—I was Nellie on "Little House on the Prairie" for seven years. My character was married off, as are all good prairie people, to Percival Dalton, played by an actor named Steve Tracy. I was actually rather afraid about getting married on the show because I played a villainess, and I didn't know what awful, hideous person they would get to marry me.

I was pleased when Steve Tracy was hired, because he was a really nice guy. And I enjoyed being his TV wife. We had a great relationship. Not everyone who gets married on TV gets along. We

157

became fast friends and went absolutely everywhere together, to the point that rumors were circulating that we were having some torrid affair. Of course, we decided to play it up all the more because he was gay and dating a guy and I was dating a guy who wasn't socially acceptable. He was too old and he had a tattoo—too terrible a person for some good, wholesome TV star to be going out with. And so we thought, well, why don't we just throw in the towel and say we're dating each other and make everybody real happy, because that's their fantasy anyway, and that's our job, to fulfill fantasies.

We stayed friends after the show. One night, he called me up and left this really weird message on my machine. I knew something was wrong. When I talked to him he told me that he had some form of cancer and that he couldn't talk about it because there were other people around. Eventually I talked to him, and it was true. He had Kaposi's sarcoma, but he didn't say that it was Kaposi's sarcoma, not that I would've known what the hell that meant at the time anyway. And he didn't say that he had AIDS either.

Later he called one afternoon to say, "Look, you know that cancer I told everyone I had? I really have to level with you—it's AIDS. I'm going on 'A.M. Los Angeles' tomorrow because I just can't stand it anymore. You know, I've never been a liar. I've never lied about being gay. It *is* AIDS."

He was telling half his friends, "I have nothing," some friends, "I have cancer," and some friends, "I have AIDS." And he said, "I can't keep my stories straight. To hell with it. Maybe it'll do some good if the guy from 'Little House on the Prairie' has this."

I was a basket case, because I loved him. He told me he had this disease, which I'd been reading killed you, and I screamed bloody murder. Not on the phone of course. I tried to be real brave, because he was being horribly brave and cheerful and tough.

When he went public, the *National Enquirer* went berserk. But one would expect, what else? It's their job. They called my house. They called my unlisted home phone number. They called my parents. They called everybody. And they asked all kinds of dopey questions. They called my parents and asked, "Well, does she have it?" All sorts of people called up going, "Well, what's up? Talk." And I would say, "Well, it's called AIDS, and he's got it. And that's all I know."

I needed to educate myself so that I could educate all these people who were asking me questions. And I needed to find out what I could do to help Steve. I started by training to be a hotline volunteer at AIDS Project Los Angeles. I remember that Steve was very pleased. He said, "Oh, yes. That's a very good thing. Yeah, you'll be good at that."

When Melissa [Gilbert] got word about Steve, she called me up and said, "Well, that's it. We're having a reunion party. This is important. One of our friends is sick. The party's at my house. Everyone is invited and they're all coming." I said, "What if anybody gives us flak?" And she said, "If anybody pulls any shit, if anybody wants to eat off of paper plates, or doesn't come, I will personally punch their lights out. They're coming to this party, and they're all going to behave themselves." So we all went to Melissa's and everybody did show up. The only people who didn't show were working on location or were sick. Michael Landon was working, but his kids, Leslie and Mike, Jr., came. They were friends of Melissa's. No one from the show rejected Steve because he had AIDS. But then we people on "Little House on the Prairie" are a cut above your average group of low-life actors, so there!

Steve was told that he had six months to live when he was diagnosed. He lived about a year and a half past when he was supposed to die. He was a long-term survivor for his day.

His death was like a large cannonball going through my stomach, passing out the other side. I was only 23 when he died and, I'm sorry, I didn't know a lot of dead people. I do now. I'm like a lot of people my age. I'm not even old enough to have known anyone who died in Vietnam. So to have a lot of people my age, friends of mine, dying, is traumatic.

A couple of years later, the press ran a lot of old photographs that they had of him and me, and I wasn't sure how to take it. I was happy for him that he got this publicity, but I cried. I called his mom and said, "Marge, what do you want me to do? Do you want me to do this? I mean, this is your son, your only son. You're his mom, for God's sake. I'm just his deadbeat friend. They want to run his picture whenever they do an article with me. They want to mention AIDS, and they want to talk about him. Does this bother you? Should I do less, more? Should I cease and desist?" And she said, "Are you kidding? Think about who we're talking about here. We're taking about a man whose ashes are scattered under the Hollywood sign." Seriously, he's under the Hollywood sign. And she said, "We're talking about a man who, on his deathbed, noticed that there was this little spotlight in the ceiling and said, 'Oh, good. A key light.'"

I think keeping Steve's memory alive is important. It is to me and to his mom and his sister. And I think it is to people with AIDS, so that they know people with AIDS are not forgotten. It is important that people remember these are people's children. This is somebody's baby, somebody's son, somebody's husband, somebody's friend.

What would I say to someone else who has a friend with AIDS?

Well, first of all, obviously, stay their friend. They need you now more than ever. I've had several friends with AIDS—all very diverse people who needed different things. Remember that if your friend has always been a proud and independent person, they won't want you to play nursemaid, no matter how sick they get. Even if they need you to, they won't want you to. Steve was a very independent person. When he was having nerve damage and would fall down, nobody was allowed to help him up. That was the thing. I could only vent my maternal instincts so far with him, because he was like, "I'll get it myself." Try to remember, don't embarrass your friends if they are sick.

How did I get through Steve's illness?

You know, we always say, "Get through it." But it's horrible and you're going to suffer, and that's all there is to it. I know that sounds terrible, but I had a friend of mine whose friend was dying and he said, "Well, what do I do? How do I deal with this?" I said, "Are you asking me to tell you some magic to make this not hurt? I have really bad news for you. There isn't something you can make happen that will make them not die. Or you think they'll die and you'll go, 'Oh, OK' and just get up and go to the funeral and then go eat lunch afterward? You think this is going to be fine? It is not fine. They're not coming to dinner anymore. They're not going to come to your house, and you can't go to the movies with them. And they won't be there when you phone them, when you have a problem and need someone to talk to. That's going to feel bad. You need to accept the fact that they are going to be gone and that you are going to hate it. There will be things you didn't say to them and you're going to beat yourself up and rip your hair out and bash your head against the wall that you never said them. You're going to regret every stupid thing you ever said to them when you were mad. But the thing is, they probably know. They probably understand."

It also helps me to know that when I do speaking engagements at schools, these kids who don't know anyone with AIDS watch "Little House" and they know Steve. And for some reason, hearing something from Nellie Olson means more to them than from a doctor. Personally, I think this is kind of stupid, that someone would get their AIDS information from Nellie Olson, but since that's the case, then fine.

I'm also involved with Tuesday's Child, which provides direct services to families with children with AIDS. I've been there full-time for the last year. We just got out our Thanksgiving baskets and Christmas baskets to all the families. And then we have our regular services, providing diapers and food and clothing and transportation—all kinds of keen stuff.

In the beginning I did it for Steve. I was doing it for me, too. My phone was ringing. People were asking questions and I didn't have the answers. I thought if they were going to be silly enough to ask, I should have something to tell them. And then after Steve there's been Jim Glove and Jim Scotland and John T. and Tom Scout and Tom Lang and so on and on and on. Tom Lang was my husband's best friend from high school. My husband has lost friends. My parents have lost a lot of theirs. And now, of course, I have the children [at Tuesday's Child], who have completely stolen my heart and ruined my life.

I'm pretty much devoting my time to AIDS. And I'm still trying to get a [television] series. But I have post-child-star syndrome. It's a bitch to get work. It's hard. You know, no one wants to hire anyone who was on a series. But if I get a series I'd be so jazzed because then I'd have more money to spend on AIDS. And I would shanghai the cast of whatever I was doing and get them involved. And I would have TV fuel to flaunt for this project.

—*ALISON ARNGRIM*

162

☐ Steve Tracy died on November 27, 1986, at age 33.

In addition to all of her other AIDS-related projects, Alison Arngrim hosts a cable television show called "AIDS Vision."

Lucille Zarse, 57, is a free-lance writer and AIDS volunteer in Lafayette, Indiana. In May 1989, she and her husband, Harold, met 37-year-old Robert Wilson. It was a meeting that would change all of their lives.

Robert had returned to his hometown to die.

I had a former employer whom I used to love dearly, and I learned that he was ill. I kept calling, asking, "What's wrong with him?" "Well," they said, "don't say anything, but he has AIDS." I said, "My God! Why? How?" "Well," they said, "blood transfusions." So when he died, that's when it really hit me and I said, "I can't stand this. I've got to do something." It started out by donation, money. We always think money can talk. It doesn't. It really doesn't even help the conscience. Because I would give money and say, "I don't feel any better." So finally I joined an organization that had this buddy program. I went into that gung-ho. You know, "Boy, I'm going to save the world!"

Anyway, I was working at a post-office job. My husband told me that somebody had called and wanted him to transport a boy with AIDS, give him rides. His balance was off and so forth and he hadn't purchased a car yet. He had returned to Lafayette from New York.

164

Later my husband kept saying things like, "Well, you ought to meet this boy. He's so nice," and so on and so forth. Then one day he said, "I'm supposed to take Robert to the doctor. I want you to come along." So I went and I thought, "Gee, you know, he is so polite and so nice." My heart went out to him. It was probably the next day. We went over to his house, and on top of his television was this beautiful lavender glass sculpture. I just went crazy over it. Robert laughed and said, "You know, you're the only other person who likes it." Well, now I have it.

As time went on, actually just a few days, we were really, really close. He had tuberculosis, pneumocystis, and Kaposi's sarcoma. But just to go over and hug him was a wonderful feeling. People can sense if you're faking it or not. He knew we weren't. I loved that boy. He was wonderful. One day I hugged him and said, "Oh, I'm in love." And he said, "Sorry, you have the wrong plumbing, my dear." I will never forget that. I thought it was so cute.

One day we were talking in the hospital and he had a terrible bout with throwing up. He said, "I hate to do that. I'm always afraid I'm going to choke to death because, you know, my mom, that's how she died." I said, real quickly, "Oh my God! She was in California. She was married to a Navy man. She had just had a baby!" He said, "You knew my mom?" I said, "Her name was Betty." I had known Betty, this would've been when Robert was a baby, because she worked as a waitress in a restaurant that I went to a lot. That's where Betty met her new husband. He married her and they moved to California, and Betty put Robert in an orphanage. Robert's real father got Robert out of the orphanage a while later, and they moved to California too, but Robert never did see his mother again. I guess Robert's father remarried and tried to make them a family again. Then, when Robert was in his early teens, he told his father that he was gay, and his father kicked him out of the house. Robert lived a very hard life from 14 on, and he never did reconcile with his father. When Robert moved back to Lafayette to die, he lived in the same apartment building as his father [who had also returned to Lafayette], but his father only went up to see him a few times, and even then he wouldn't say much, just "hi," and then leave.

But I think it comforted Robert that I knew his mother. When we talked about her, he would smile. I told him he looked like her, and he smiled when I said that. He asked me what she was like—was she pretty? Of course I said yes, because she really was an attractive woman. Plus I think every child wants to think or does think that his mother is beautiful. He had a lot of mixed feelings about her, his whole family. We really only talked about his mother in detail that one day, but it was like our little special connection. In a way it made us closer. I had known Betty, and now I was taking care of her son.

If I were a real religious person I'd probably say that God spoke to me. But no one spoke to me. It was just like, *this is it!* I decided to quit my job at the post office to take care of Robert. I thought, I'm going to give him so much love, so much caring, that he won't even realize that he has such a short time.

We met Robert in May of 1989, and he died—or as I'd rather state, he went beyond his form, on September 7 of that year. And during that time, we lived his life with him. We spent a portion of each day with him. We shopped with him, dined with him, we, the three of us, were absolutely crazy together on his "good days." And on his bad days, one of just held him and comforted him and stayed with him as long as seven hours at a time.

But there were happy times, too, and they far outweighed the sad. For example, our constant rivalry to outdo one another in the area of the great classics, our uncontrollable urge to gorge ourselves on cinnamon candy, our love of the color purple, and the contests we engaged in to prove that one of us possessed more items of that color than the other.

It was if I had gone through a gate and couldn't go back and be the person I had been before. We all fall into this trap of flailing around about how this isn't fair. You know, "Why did they do this?" And suddenly, it hit me, the last time Robert was in the hospital. Why waste your energy when we have a young person up here who should be living 50 more years and he's dying? I have to save my energy to look after him.

There were times when I wondered, Am I his caretaker or is he my mentor? What a teacher he was!

I was never a very physical person. Robert enabled me to comfortably touch and hug, and I found myself doing this to many friends, relatives, and acquaintances.

He amazed me with his positive outlook and uplifting personality, while at the same time I knew that he was aware of his prognosis. He was indeed a tough fighter, and I believe he felt that this disease wasn't going to conquer him, most assuredly he would win! I wasn't privileged to have known him as the healthy person he had been before AIDS. I only saw the Kaposi's sarcoma, the weakened body, the frail, gentle person scarred by the disease during his last four and a half months. I became aware of his courage, warmth, the tenderness, the rebel, and, in his eyes, the person he had been before the disease.

As the tumor in his brain progressed, he lost his speech, yet he always had a smile for us, and he'd look directly into our eyes. He could only say a few swear words, which livened up so many so-called one-sided conversations. His specialty was "shit" and "damn!" These words were so endearing to me because they were all he could say, and he so needed to express himself. Harold, my partner and best friend, seemed to be able to detect exactly what

Robert was wanting without any difficulty. And he was so patient with him.

By August 25, Robert became comatose, although he'd cough occasionally. We knew he was leaving his form, still, he was on massive amounts of morphine. By September 3, Robert was diagnosed with tubercular pneumonia, and he responded to nothing. On September 7, at 12:00 A.M., Robert died.

He was a gay proud gentleman.

I felt no regrets in my relationship with and care of him.

Everything that you are ultimately wears out and dies, but thought *never* dies. He went beyond his form.

Robert taught us how to hope and love, how to win and how to lose. He taught us how to live, and finally, he taught us how to die.

—LUCILLE ZARSE

I decided to do what I love best—sing and dance.

Since my diagnosis of Kaposi's sarcoma and AIDS in December 1988, I've only been sick twice. Both times have been in the spring. In April of 1990 and 1991, I came down with high fevers and fatigue and lost about 15 pounds. Both times the doctors couldn't diagnose what I had. I was sick for about a month each time, and then whatever it was just went away and I was fine. The doctors gave me anti-inflammatories each time, and that seemed to do the trick.

I started on AZT in January of 1989 and was on it for two years with no problems. But it was losing its effect, so in February 1991 I started on DDI and have had no problems with it. And since my diagnosis of KS in 1988, I went through six weeks of mild chemotherapy, and that seemed to arrest the KS. I've had no new lesions.

When I got sick the second time, in April of 1991, I decided to quit work [at the gym] because I just couldn't do it anymore. I needed to concentrate on my health. Since that time, I've been on disability.

I've changed certain things in my life since I was diagnosed, but for the most part, I've always led a pretty healthy life. I've worked out at least three days a week, sometimes five days a week, for the past 10 years. In addition to quitting my job, I stopped partying, stopped hanging out in the clubs, and I've been in a relationship with the same person for over two years. It's the longest relationship I've ever had with a man.

But the thing that has made me the happiest, the thing that has done the most for my spirit has been going back to my first love—the theater. When I was growing up in Georgia, I was always doing community theater, and I was involved in theater at school, but I had let it go for the past three or four years. In March of 1991 I tried out for a workshop production of a show called *Dirty Dreams of a Clean-Cut Kid*, but I got sick and couldn't perform. Later a guy dropped out of the show, and the writer called me up, and all of a sudden I was working in a cabaret show. It was a dream come true.

The show is about four guys waiting for the results of their AIDS tests at a clinic. All the characters sing, and the story could be mine, yours, anybody's. I love it. It really gives me something to stay healthy for and to fight for. It gives me another reason to live. I get to touch people when I'm on stage and with this show. I can also give them a message. The message is "Get tested. Don't wait. Do it now. And then you can start to live your life in a way that's best for you."

I met my lover when I knew I was HIV-positive. He had been tested but hadn't gotten the results back yet. When they came back positive, it didn't matter to either one of us. We wanted to have a life together. And so we started our lives over. And even though I have AIDS, I feel that I'm lucky. Rick and I have each other. I have a supportive family, and I'm doing what makes me the happiest in the world, I'm entertaining. I wanted to be a part of the entertainment industry all my life. I thought when I was diagnosed that the dream was over. But I find now that it's not over, that it's only begun. Even though I have AIDS, the show must go on.

—BUDDY MONTGOMERY

☐ Buddy Montgomery is 31 years old. As of this writing Buddy is still relatively healthy and still entertaining. Buddy's goal is to take his show on the road. Says he, "I want my legacy to be more than a Yugo and a Judy Garland collection."

I got an HIV test in Portland and then went to San Francisco for a vacation to wait out the results. I needed to pull myself away from the situation and examine it before I went back to face the doctor.

The test came back positive.

That's when I met Buddy Montgomery. We met at the gym in San Francisco when he was working the desk. He asked me to lunch, and at lunch he told me about himself, that he was HIV-positive and everything. I told him that I hadn't gotten the test results back yet, but that I expected them to be positive.

Buddy's been a good coach for me. He had been diagnosed with AIDS a year before me. And we hit it off. I think the fact that we were both facing the AIDS crisis actually drew us together. That, as well as being attracted to each other and liking the other's mind and strengths and whatnot. We've both just crossed 30, and we're starting to become more down-to-earth, more domestic. This has been the best relationship in my whole gay life.

Anyway, I decided to move to San Francisco from Portland, not only because of Buddy but also because of the openness and because of all the health programs. I just feel a lot more supported here than I would have in Portland.

I quit smoking. I quit doing drugs, other than what I have to take for my epilepsy, which I have because of a motorcycle accident four years ago. I don't smoke pot. And I don't drink at all. I work out. I'm very avid about working out. For me, it's good mentally and physically. My main social life has been going to the gym and working out.

What would I say to others?

Well, I've encountered people who have this attitude of, I'm positive; I'm going to die anyway, so I might as well live it up while it lasts. I don't think that's the best approach at all. All you're going to do is cut your life short. I think you need to make the best of each day. Why say to yourself, Well, I'm going to die anyway, when you could say, Well, I'm going to live; *while I'm living, I'm going to live?*

—*RICK WRIGHT*

☐ Rick Wright, 34, tested HIV-positive in September 1989. As of this writing he is still in a relationship with Buddy Montgomery and had registered to go back to school.

As the chair of the Senate Subcommittee on Disability Policy, I had the distinct privilege of meeting Belinda Mason when she testified during the consideration of the Americans with Disabilities Act of 1990. Belinda Mason was a young journalist from Tobinsport, Indiana, who tested positive for the HIV virus in March of 1987. Rather than give in to self-pity, Belinda became an advocate for persons with AIDS and served as a board member of the National Association of People with AIDS.

Even though Belinda contracted the AIDS virus through a blood transfusion, she understood that the HIV disease is blind to race, age, gender, and sexual orientation. She testified that those with AIDS are "just like us because they *are* us."

My thoughts upon Belinda's death were of her husband and two small children and the inestimable cost of AIDS to our society. But I also remember Belinda's courage in the face of adversity and her commitment to ending discrimination. Belinda described the discrimination she experienced and related that she found that America is "not a good place to be different or ill."

When I think of Belinda, I remember the moving statement she made about the discrimination faced by those associated with AIDS in her testimony before the subcommittee:

> With [the HIV-positive] diagnosis, I became a person with a hidden disability, a disability just like epilepsy and diabetes and tens of other hidden disabilities. And just like people with those other hidden disabilities, I became the subject of irrational and unjustified discrimination. . . . When we look in the mirror that AIDS and HIV holds up to society, we see how scared we are of each other, of death, and even life. We can see how little tolerance, let along compassion, that we often show.

Belinda will be missed both personally and in the fight to secure compassionate treatment for persons who are HIV-positive or have AIDS. But she left behind a legacy—her commitment to the goal of eliminating discrimination against persons with AIDS and those associated with them.

Because of Belinda and advocates like her, discrimination is now illegal. The Americans with Disabilities Act of 1990 provides recourse for those who are discriminated against and, as Belinda stated, provides the legislative support necessary to "help promote reason and foster more decent treatment."

—*SEN. TOM HARKIN*

I make it through each day by staying busy. Since I had to quit work [in hotel management], I now have a lot of time on my hands. So I try to keep busy. Some people tell me that's denial. I say, "So what?" It works for me.

I wake up at seven every morning, and then I make a schedule for myself for the whole day. No matter how little something may seem, I include it in my schedule. I even treat mailing a letter like a big event. I spend a lot of time with my friends who really help me stay "up." I laugh a lot and am very positive in my thinking.

Up until two months ago I hadn't been to church in over 20 years. But one of my friends talked me into going to a gay church service, and it has changed my life. I have a lot of hope that I am going to survive this disease, but if I don't, I have belief in God. I believe that there's someplace to go once I leave this earth. Everyone has to believe in something, and believing in the afterlife is the one thing that gets me through each day. I feel that it's very important for me to be in touch with my spiritual self, and church has put me in touch with that part of me I thought was gone. I find great joy and comfort in believing that I will go on.

When I was first diagnosed, I thought, I'm going to kill myself and get it over with. I don't want to suffer or put my family and friends through this. But my family and friends told me that they would be with me every step of the way—and they have been.

To me, support groups were depressing, but I know that they work for some people. Church is my support group, and it has taught me to have hope and not to give up. I will never lie in bed and feel sorry for myself. I won't give up, because I have so much to live for. I am going to travel and experience as much as I can.

—ANTHONY RIVIERA

☐ Anthony Riviera is 36 years old. He was diagnosed with Kaposi's sarcoma and AIDS in August 1988. His health has since fluctuated up and down. His spirits, ebullient and inspiring, remarkably have not.

Carol Lynn and Gerald Pearson were married in the Salt
Lake City Temple in 1966. Despite membership in the
Mormon church, they divorced 12 years and four
children later when they both realized that Gerald's
homosexual proclivities were not a frivolous or passing
fancy. He moved out of the family home in Walnut
Creek, California, and into an apartment in San
Francisco.

For the next six years they struggled to rebuild their
individual lives while also maintaining their friendship
and some semblance of family.

Gerald would return to Walnut Creek for family
activities. Carol Lynn would go to San Francisco and
meet Gerald's boyfriends.

Their marriage started out in storybook fashion, but
their relationship after the divorce broke all traditional
standards and spoke volumes about their resolve and
spirit and unconditional love.

And then, in March 1984, Carol Lynn received a phone
call from Gerald. It was a call that she had feared.
"Blossom [his longtime pet name for her]," he said, "I
have AIDS."

Carol Lynn responded by welcoming her former
husband back into the same Walnut Creek home that he
had left six years before. She, along with their children,

watched over Gerald, participated in his laugh therapy (the children would collect all the jokes they heard at school and pass them on to their father), and encouraged and comforted him, all the while hoping for a miracle recovery.

A couple of days after the diagnosis, Gerald just sat down with the children upstairs in my bedroom and told them he was sick. He told them that he needed their support and help and that he was determined to get better. I saw some tears that day. The children had had classes in school about AIDS. They all knew about it.

Gerald had pneumonia. He was put into the hospital immediately. He recovered and maintained his health for a bit after that, determined to keep on living. He could not believe that the end of his life was imminent. He had a lot of things still to accomplish, a lot of things still to resolve. He knew that he had not succeeded very well in his adventures of going out, trying to make it work in the gay community. He was very proud of some of the things he had done, like his work in the Gay Men's Chorus, but he had not succeeded in establishing a lasting relationship with somebody he loved. And he very much wanted to see our children grow older.

"I expected Gerald to pull off a miracle. In spite of everything we had been through, in spite of all the confusions and problems, I continued to see something in Gerald that to me was almost supernatural. I kept a romanticized view of him even though the romance was gone. His gifts were so good. His desire to do something helpful was so deep. . . .

"I developed a fantasy and held on to it

179

determinedly. Gerald would get well. . . . He would be
the bridge he had so wanted to be to develop
understanding of homosexuals to the larger world. . . .
He had often quoted someone who said, 'Most men
die with their music still in them.' Gerald had sung,
but not all his songs. Not all! Surely there would be a
miracle!"

—CAROL LYNN PEARSON

There was this undercurrent of guilt that I suppose everyone gets after being told all your life by society that your basic inner core is wrong. And even if you spend years getting away from that, when something dreadful happens, you cannot help but say, "Were they right after all?" I'm sure those thoughts went through Gerald's head, but he quickly threw them out. I know he was battling some things about the [Mormon] church. He was going through meditation and affirmations to free him from these things, these tapes that were in his mind.

After I let the church group know what was happening to Gerald, they came to the house and were very quick to say, "What can we do for you?" I asked the Women's Auxiliary president [of the church] and her husband if they could find someone from the church I could pay to do some cleaning up. It had been a couple of months, and the yard was just a mess. But one day *they*, along with their one son, came over and spent the whole day working in my yard. It was a major, major cleanup. Other members of the church brought over various things and made other kinds of phone calls for me. And my own divinity teacher called and said, "I'm not going to say, 'Let me know if you need anything.' That's not good enough. I want you to make a list of all the things you need to have taken care of, and I'm going to call you every morning at nine o'clock and you can tell me all the things that need to be done. And we'll go do them."

> *"People who won't even drink coffee have a hard time*
> *understanding homosexuality and AIDS, but they*
> *don't have a hard time understanding suffering and*
> *need."*
>
> —CAROL LYNN PEARSON

I suppose I had some faith that this would all make sense some-where, sometime. I did believe that there was some eternal picture. I certainly, you know, had faith that doing the best we could for one another was the only way to go about living life. And I certainly felt comfortable that I was doing what I could for Gerald—and that is important to know. Something else that has always been helpful to me was keeping a diary since high school.

Gerald had been staying at home alone while I was on vacation with the kids. When we walked in that door at about 10 o'clock at night after having been gone for a week, I was just astonished to see how far he had gone down. The children were shocked. He was sitting up on the black couch in his blue bathrobe, waiting for his family to come back. He had shaved off his beard. He looked very wasted. After having to see that, as I was getting the other kids off to bed, Emily, the oldest, went out onto the porch and started sobbing. I went out to sit with her, and she said, "Mom, he's already dead."

It was an extremely painful thing to see this man who had been so full of life and ambition and warmth just waste away in front of me. I had maintained a lot of affection for him even after we had ended the marriage, and it hardly seemed possible to me that he had this *thing* and was moving toward his death. Intellectually, I knew it was happening, but emotionally, it was very hard to deal with.

I put him in the hospital the next day for a blood transfusion, which pepped him up a little bit.

> *"Are you watching the news, Blossom? Geraldine Ferraro won the vice-presidential nomination. Isn't that great?"*
>
> *"Actually, Gerald, I haven't had time to even think about it."*
>
> *"Well, take the time. Celebrate a little!"*
>
> **—GERALD AND CAROL LYNN**
> in a telephone call made by
> Gerald from his hospital bed

There was nothing else the hospital could do for him, so I just brought him home. The next few days told me that he was going to go rapidly. I was determined to let him stay home without putting him back into the hospital or any other kind of facility. And then Gerald died. I'm glad that it all happened quite rapidly. You know, by the time he started to go down, it went very fast. I didn't have a lot of time to think. It was July 1984.

What would I say to someone else going through a similar experience?

If I had harbored a lot of hatred for Gerald, I think it would have made the whole thing even harder. Maybe not everyone would agree with this, but I think to give up somebody you love is a lot easier than to give up somebody you hate, because there is such a lot of unsettled stuff there. Gerald and I had settled most of our stuff. And that was helpful to me.

None of us is going to get out of this world scot-free. Every one of us is going to, in one way or another, go through what these people were going through. For some of us, it will be long and agonizing. For some of us, it will be quick. All of us are going to be faced with exactly what they are facing. And so we don't for a minute need to think that these guys are getting it and the rest of us aren't. We're *all* going to get it.

The highest law is the law of love and compassion.

—CAROL LYNN PEARSON

☐ After her former husband's death, Carol Lynn Pearson, a 51-year-old poet and performer, wrote her autobiography, *Good-bye, I Love You.* It was adapted in part from her diaries written during the course of her husband's illness.

At the time of this writing she is touring with a one-woman play that she wrote and was performing. "Gerald," says Carol Lynn, "would be thrilled about the play." He would be thrilled, too, that his songs are still being sung.

I always try to look for any good I can find in a situation and make the best of it. I have a value for life now that I didn't have before. Valued life. Valued friends. I didn't have much of a focus before, either. Now I have a focus: I'm fighting for my life.

I believe that I am not going to die a day sooner than I was intended to. Regardless of whether I have 20 days or 20 years, *I don't want to die before I'm dead.* I want to live before I die.

If I could say something to the world, it would be this: Don't think that it couldn't happen to you, because it can. I was a nice, Protestant white boy. I didn't think that something like this could happen to me. And it did.

—*ROGER DUNCAN*

☐ **Roger Duncan was 37 years old when he was stricken with pneumonia and diagnosed with AIDS in January 1990. He has since traveled frequently to and from his present and past homes in Los Angeles and Tampa, respectively.**

   His childhood ambition was to be a psychologist. His present ambition is to see a Democrat in the White House.

On October 13, 1983, three-year-old Samuel Kushnick died of AIDS, which he had contracted through a blood transfusion received at birth.

Recently, Samuel's twin sister, Sara, wrote a poem to help her get through the ordeal. We thank Sara and her mother, Helen Gorman Kushnick, Jay Leno's manager, for allowing us to reprint Sara's poem below.

Today Sara, 11, attends sixth grade in the Los Angeles area. It is Sara's hope that her poem will help others who are losing loved ones to AIDS.

DEATH

By Sara R. Kushnick

When there is death in your life,
your balloons start to drop.

When you go outside to play
instead of a hop, you walk.

Your tears are sour, not like before
when you just hear about it
you don't feel any more.

You scream out loud, "No!"
to show your grief,
you think life is a thief.

You sit and weep
you think life is a mountain
too hard to climb, too steep.

You have thoughts
you just can't bottle up inside.

Let them out if you have a doubt
Let them out if there's something
you need to talk about.

*I*n New York in the early 1980s hemophiliacs were concerned about the blood supply because of the AIDS epidemic. Then, in 1983, the doctor I went to told all of us [hemophiliacs] to just assume that we were HIV-positive, but because there was not any kind of treatment yet not to bother being tested. In 1985 we were advised by our doctor to get tested, and I did. I was positive. I was 23 years old at the time.

My T-cells were considered good, over 300 at the time, and in 1985 people weren't put on AZT until they went below 200 T-cells. So from 1985 to 1987 I was without any kind of treatment. When my T-cells dropped to 36, I started the early dosage of AZT of two capsules five times a day—a total of 10 AZT a day. I became horribly sick. I couldn't open my eyes. I couldn't drive. I could barely move. It was just horrible. It is the sickest I have ever been since I tested positive. And it wasn't because of the AIDS; it was because of the AZT.

I dropped my dosage of AZT to one, five times a day and was on it for a year and a half, but then I just couldn't take it anymore. It wasn't working for me anymore, and my T-cells were continually dropping. For six months I wasn't on anything and felt great. I had no symptoms of AIDS. In April of 1990 I started on DDI and was only on it for four months when I developed a severe side effect called neuropathy. I lost the feeling in my hands and feet. It was horribly debilitating for me. I was taking one dose every 12 hours. I stopped the DDI. In 1990 I also started taking aerosolized pentamidine so that I wouldn't develop pneumocystis carinii pneumonia. I do that treatment about once a month, and it has had no adverse effects on me so far. I didn't take any kind of antiviral medication from April 1990 until March 1991. In March of 1991 I started taking DDC and was only on that for two months before I started getting horrible red blotches and rashes all over my body, in addition to neuropathy. So I went off DDC in May 1991 and am currently not taking anything. All the medications that I took made me sicker than the AIDS.

In September 1990 I was diagnosed with full-blown AIDS. The signs of toxoplasmosis started in early August of 1990—severe headaches. I had a lot of CAT scans, but nothing showed up. It wasn't until I switched doctors and he gave me an MRI [Magnetic Resonance Imaging] that he discovered an enormous amount of toxo, on my brain. It was full-blown toxo! I was very lucky. I had no neurological damage. I have recovered from this bout with toxo and am currently doing fine. I get tired easily and don't have a lot of stamina, but I really haven't had a bad illness in six years except for the toxo.

After the toxo I was told my T-cells had dropped to six—that was in September 1990. But I have lived with those six T-cells for a year, and I'm still going strong. The toxo never leaves, but with treatment it is under control. I should be dead with the amount of toxo that I had in my brain, but I'm too mean to die. I've kept my weight at 165, so I've had no problem with weight loss. I was normally about 175 to 180, but when I had toxo, I lost some weight. I just look better with it off, so I have chosen to keep it off.

In some ways I think that we hemophiliacs who contracted AIDS were actually more prepared for the illness. We grew up used to having illnesses, used to spending time in hospitals, and used to seeing our doctors on a very regular basis, unlike the general population, who goes to a doctor once or twice a year, if even that.

I lost a lot of my younger years to illness, so this is really nothing new to me—to lose a week by having the flu or something or to spend time in the house resting. I think it's almost easier for me to accept, in that regard, because I was never 100 percent healthy in my life. So I guess I didn't have as much to lose as other people did.

Growing up, I learned to compartmentalize my illness. I deal with it when I'm not feeling well, and I don't think about it when I feel healthy. So my pattern hasn't changed a lot since I've had AIDS. I treat my AIDS the same way I treat my hemophilia.

I came to Los Angeles from New York in 1989 to go to graduate school at Pepperdine University to become an attorney, but I just didn't have the energy or strength to put in 60 hours a week to study. So I've had to change my direction a bit, and now I own a recording studio. I rent it out and produce demos for bands, but right now I'm really not doing very much. As strong as I think I am and as full a life as I lead, I'm the first to admit that I don't have the energy of my peers. This noticeable decrease in energy has happened in the past three years. I mean, at my age men are at their partying prime. It was taking me longer and longer to recoup the next day. I don't have the ability to work eight or nine hours a day and then go out and party at night as my friends do. I've reached a point when I cannot work *and* play. If I want to go out at night

189

and have a drink, one for each of my six T-cells, I stay home and rest during the day. I was supposed to go back to graduate school in September 1990, but I came down with the toxo, and now I just don't have the energy to go back. My friends think that I'm lazy and unambitious. I haven't told a lot of my friends I have AIDS.

As much as the hemophilia may make it easier for me to accept having AIDS on a physical level, my heterosexuality has made it much more difficult for me to accept than if I were homosexual. I think that the heterosexual community is very ignorant in a lot of ways about the risk of AIDS and about the people who have it. From what I know from my friends who are homosexual, homosexuals just accept that a person they are interested in dating is either HIV-positive or is at least aware that he could be. And if they are or aren't positive, homosexual men are aware and educated enough to practice safe sex. Straight people, especially young straight men, don't think they can get AIDS, and for the most part they don't practice safe sex. From what I've experienced, straight people will not ask [your HIV status]. You have to tell them, and when you do, it's much harder for them to accept. In the gay community everyone is at least aware of the possibility, and if someone is HIV-positive or has AIDS, you can still start a new relationship. In the straight community that's almost impossible.

I was single when I was told I was HIV-positive. Since then I have dated, and when I tell the girls, well, they just can't handle it. It didn't bother one girl, but her friends kept telling her to drop me because there are so many healthy men in the world, why should she risk her life with me? So she left under their pressure.

But in many, many ways I am very lucky. I have a strong support system with my family. I have a really good doctor, Michael Roth. And I have a very good psychologist who helps me work out a lot of things, my anger and my fears. I believe in God. I don't necessarily believe in any kind of church, but I believe that there is a God up there and that He has some kind of plan in mind for everyone. He didn't just put us all here to suffer.

I try to exercise and relax with the world. For me, I find the water, the beach, very relaxing, so I live at the beach. It impresses me so much to see the power of nature. It makes me feel that human life is so much smaller than the big world around it and that our problems aren't that big.

People die so easily and quickly in accidents or car wrecks without even thinking about it [death]. At least I can think about it, plan it, have an option. I've been fortunate in that I am allowed to focus my life on just staying well. I look to the future. I don't make just short-term goals, I make long-term goals. As long as I can recover from my illnesses and still be myself and not a shadow of myself, life is worth living.

—*WILLIAM O'BRIEN**

☐ The preceding interview with William O'Brien took place in September 1991. He died in December at the age of 28.

*This name is an alias. The parents of "William O'Brien" made no mention of AIDS in their son's obituary and have insisted that his real name not be mentioned in these pages.

❏ ❏

*H*ello, my name is Iris. I am a very grateful recovering alcoholic and addict. I am 38 years old and have an 18-year-old son. I found out on February 26, 1991, that I had full-blown AIDS, with 20 T-cells. It blew me away.

When I was 13, I was beaten, raped, dragged into an alley, and hung by my panties and bra. I was unconscious for 28 days. But I lived. It was then that my mother's preacher told me that God must have a plan for me. Now I know what that plan is. You see, teenagers don't like to be told what to do and what not to do. But they see me, clean and sober after 23 years of drug abuse, and they say, "Hey, if she can do it, I can, too." They see me, fat, fine, healthy, and clean, and they say, "Hey, Iris looks good. If she can do it . . ."

And I talk to them about AIDS. I had gone to the doctor because the lymph nodes in my neck were large, and I also had a bad case of thrush. I was seven months pregnant at the time, and they were trying to get me to take this test, this AIDS test. I remember I kept on telling those people, "I do not want to take that test today! I won't take it!" I knew I had AIDS.

The first thing I thought when I found out was, "Oh, f—k! I can't ever have sex again!"

Now I have safe sex. Before, when I was having sex with somebody I dug, who dug me, I didn't see any reason for condoms, because I thought, This person ain't got nothing. That's what my head would tell me. But now I realize that I can't think like that, you know? Now, if I've got you in bed, you've got to get tested.

How has my life changed since I was told I had AIDS?

I realized that I could not do the same things. I could not live in the same place. I could not run around with the same people, because most of them had been addicts. I had to change my lifestyle. I had to get new friends. I had to get clean friends. I had to run with the winners.

Now I try to carry the message as best I can: *This shit is for real.* It's an equal-opportunity disease, and it kills.

—IRIS CROUCH

☐ As of this writing Iris has been stricken with pneumocystis, toxoplasmosis, CMV-retinitis, yeast infections, and seizures. Yet she is still relatively healthy and is still spreading her message of hope and education: "Fight AIDS, not people with AIDS."

Iris's childhood ambition was to open up an auto mechanics garage with her two brothers. It was to be called Crouch, Crouch and Crouch.

193

On Christmas Eve 1985, Steven Paul received a long-distance phone call from his former lover in Los Angeles, Will Taylor. It was a phone call that would change Steven's life. Will told Steven that he had tested HIV-positive. A few days later Steven too tested positive.
     And then their love story *really* began.

Will called. This was one of those times when we were actually speaking. I thought to myself, Oh, great, like I'm really up for this. But when I spoke to Will, he said, "This isn't a social call. I just wanted to tell you that I am HIV-positive, and chances are, with the kind of sex we had, you had better go and get yourself tested." So I wandered the streets the following day. That was quite a Christmas, especially being my first Christmas alone. I wasn't terrified, but of course I couldn't get it out of my mind. I was very lucky. I had a friend who was seeing one of the top specialists at NYU [New York University], and they were starting to do experimental tests at the time. I went in and got tested. It was positive. My counts were very high at the time, so I couldn't be part of their program. But it enabled me to be tested every four to six months as part of their study. I was very lucky to have that kind of monitoring of my blood,

194

because I was very broke at the time. I couldn't afford a sandwich, yet I could go in and get all of this expensive blood work done.

Will Taylor was a landscape architect living in Los Angeles. He had to be around greenery. His hands always had to be in soil. That was such a great side of him. I learned so much from him about plants and gardening. He was always following his spiritual path, even from our first days together. It was hard for me at first because he was very home-oriented. He just loved sitting back, making meals, playing in the garden. I loved all that stuff, but there was also a part of me that wanted the action. I had never had *my* time. I was a very straight kid. I didn't even have a drink until I was 23, so I had some living to do. So, going to New York, I was able to get that out of my system.

Once I knew he was positive and he knew I was positive, we kept in touch and saw each other quite a bit over the next 18 months. I still lived in New York, and he lived in Los Angeles. But after 18 months of that, I decided to move back to L.A. to be with Will. Six months later he was diagnosed with thrush, and his T-cells dropped rather quickly. They had been up in the 600 to 700 range, and they dropped below 200. This was in 1987. So he started on AZT, and that worked well for about a year.

Nothing really happened during that year. Will never really changed that much about his life once he was diagnosed. He didn't have much to change. He always ate healthy, he worked out, he didn't do drugs, but he did like to drink. So he cut back on his drinking because it just didn't seem to jibe with the AZT. He was always taking herbs and vitamins, and he was always in bed every night by 10. At first that had been one of the things about Will that drove me crazy. He led a very clean life.

The first year that I moved back to L.A. we took a trip to Hawaii. Actually, Will took his whole family. He really wanted his father to see Hawaii, so we flew them over to join us for a few weeks. When we got there, Will just wasn't feeling well, and he coughed up this huge *thing*. It looked like something out of *Alien*. He started feeling very sick. A couple months later, while we were still in Kauai, after his family had arrived, he woke up in the middle of the night with a high fever, 107, and was in convulsions. So we rushed him to the other side of the island. We really didn't know what kind of treatment he would get. We were afraid they might treat him like a leper. But, thank God, there was a wonderful doctor who put his hands all over Will, just a wonderful, giving doctor. They ran a series of tests on him, and he started to feel better in the hospital. They gave him a lot of antibiotics and released him.

Will felt great for the next few weeks. But once we got back home they ran more tests on him. Six months later we found out that he had bone-marrow cancer. That's why he had the high fevers. From that point on it seemed as if he couldn't get on top of things. Once he would start to feel better, he would get hit with something else. He had pneumocystis four times. He was on aerosolized pentamidine, but it just wasn't working. Nothing was. He stopped taking AZT. DDI and DDC weren't yet available. Then he was diagnosed with CMV-retinitis, and he lost the sight in one of his eyes. He was giving himself infusions twice a day, every day, through a Hickman catheter that was surgically implanted in his chest. When he was too ill to do it, I did.

I think it was the CMV that finally got him. It was in his brain. It was everywhere. Near the end he was hearing all kinds of voices in his head, and it would drive him crazy. He couldn't turn them off. There was always a conversation going on in his head.

The last two weeks, he developed an infection in his catheter line. They tried to treat him for that, but they couldn't figure out what was causing all the pain in his head. They had all sorts of specialists, but with that, and with all the medications, they just couldn't ease the pain, they just couldn't ease the pain. Finally they injected a painkiller. Within one minute I saw the relief on his face. The pain stopped and the voices stopped, and I knew that he finally had relief. The day I brought him home from the hospital, they gave him a walker to walk with around the ward. I walked with him, and as we turned around the corner, everyone was standing and cheering for him, *Rocky*-style.

That was the last time he was on his feet. Once he came home, he was bedridden.

We brought him home to die. He was ready to take off. We had so many talks where he would just weep. He had been such an active guy, and he just couldn't take any more days of just sitting on the couch and looking out the window. He would tell me, "I'm ready, I'm ready. This isn't for me." He was really thinking of taking his own life at that time. He didn't want to waste away to 30 pounds. He wanted to split. It was so hard for him to be dependent.

At the end he had lost weight, but he didn't have that zombie look. He still had rosy cheeks. The last time I gave him a bath, he looked at his stomach and said, "I've got to start my abdominal work again. Look at my stomach. It's gotten flabby!"

During his last days, all of his family came down and stayed in our house. They were all fundamentalists. But I lived with Will, I was intimate with him, and I knew *how* he wanted to take off. I was going to honor that no matter what. On Will's last trip to his hometown in Michigan, Mark, one of his younger brothers, told Will that he didn't feel sorry for him, that he was getting everything he deserved because he was gay. At the time, his brother's wife was pregnant and would not stay in the house with Will.

So when Will was dying at home, his family came. His younger brother showed up and walked into our house. He walked by Will's bed a couple of times, but he didn't acknowledge Will. He said "hi" to everyone else, but he ignored Will—in our house! He didn't acknowledge me, either. So finally I walked up to him, put my hand out, and said, "Welcome to our home." and he said, "Yeah, yeah." Finally, someone told Will that Mark was there. Will opened his eyes and looked up and said, "Step closer, Mark; I can't see you. No, closer; you know I have only one eye." Mark was all smiles and finally got closer and closer. And then Will kicked him as hard as he could and said, "Get out of my house, you f—ing asshole!" His brother stormed out of the house. I was so proud of Will; he had gotten it out of his system.

The next day Mark came back and went into the house, and he and Will talked for 20 minutes and made their peace. Each family member spent time alone with Will. One thing I stopped was the family trying to pray over him in a circle. Will didn't want that, so I refused to let them do it. I knew what Will wanted, and that wasn't it.

In those last days Will's best friend and soul mate, Karen Fell, spoke to her guru. He told her to tell Will that when he does take off, he will see light coming from many passages and that he should go into the brightest light at the end of the tunnel. He also said that Will would hear wailing but that once he got into the light, he could only turn around for a brief second before taking off into it.

Once everyone in his family had time alone with Will, I asked him if he was ready to go, and he shook his head no. I tried to let him know that I would be all right. Will was worried that I wouldn't be able to take care of myself, and so my last words to him were, "Will, when you're ready to take off, don't worry about me. I'll be OK. When you're ready, just take off." Karen told me that when the spirit leaves the body, it goes through the top of the head and that sometimes it has trouble finding its way. The way to help is to direct it to the scalp. So I got a hairbrush and I started to gently comb Will's hair. He started to take off, and then I heard this person wailing. It was me. It was like an animal coming from the pit of my stomach. Will heard me wailing and came back into his body and opened his eyes. Karen said to him, "No, Will, take off. You are the light, you are the love. Steven will be fine. Now, take off." And he did.

At that moment, I felt such euphoria. No drug had ever made me feel so good. I made it around the bed to hug his family and cry with them. By the time I got to Karen, we hugged and then we just started to laugh because we felt that we had done it. We had helped Will take off the way he had wanted. And then I got my dogs and ran up into the hills. His family was still at the house, and I needed to be alone.

What would I say to others?

There's nothing to be afraid of. As much as we fear moving on, there's really, truly, *nothing* to be afraid of. And this is so simple: When you get down to it, it's the love you give to others that counts. Just be there. Be at their side to help them through the hard times. That's truly a joyous feeling. There were moments of joy with Will right up until his last breath. The sharing, crying, laughing are there until the end. I'm just so glad that I was a part of his life and that I was able to help him when he needed me most. Get rid of the fear in your life. Get rid of the fear of the disease and of death.

What got me through this?

His love. And knowing that I'll see him again. I don't expect to see Will's little blond face again, but I just know that at some point in the game I will see him again. My soul will move on. That's one thing in this life that I know, and Will felt the same way. I knew that this wasn't the end of Will Taylor. I knew that moving on would be blissful and joyous, and that got me through it. And I hope that one day Will will come back and get me as well. I hope that he will be my guide, my spiritual hand.

And then there was his courage. I have one more thing to tell you about Will's courage. I guess it was about a month before Will became homebound. I was going to work, running home, cooking dinner, going to the store, and trying to fit in a workout at the gym three days a week. One night I walked into the gym and there was Will, waiting for me. He wanted to work out. So Will said he would take an aerobics class while I went upstairs to work out. But I couldn't keep my mind on working out, so I went downstairs and watched Will through the glass. He didn't see me, but I just cried. I was so proud of him for his courage. He was very sick and could barely move, but he was in the back of the class, trying to move his arms and legs, and it was the kind of class where everyone is jumping all over the place. Then he wanted to take a shower. I mean, he had a Hickman hanging out of his chest and his body was a mere half of what it used to be, and he was taking a shower with these guys who looked like gods. He asked me, "Do you think the guys will mind if I take a shower with my catheter in?" I said, "No, I will be there with you." We took a shower, and that kind of courage made me cry as I followed him home in my car. That was the last time he ever went to the gym.

—STEVEN PAUL

☐ Will Taylor died on August 25, 1990, at the age of 36. As of this writing Steven Paul, 36, is still working, still healthy, and still running through the hills with his—and Will's—dogs.

Brenda Freiberg, 53, has had not one but *two* sons stricken with HIV. Brett died in March 1991 at the age of 29. As of this writing her other son, Michael, 27, has yet to come down with a serious AIDS-related infection but is struggling with a T-cell count of about 100.

As a mother of two gay sons, AIDS was obviously something that I'd been afraid of. The night Brett told me that he was HIV-positive was like my worst fears realized. I think I was almost in a daze. I couldn't believe it. I couldn't believe it.

Brett was very, very aggressive with traditional Western medicine. He went on AZT long before it was approved. He took everything. He had MAI. What he really died from, though, was Kaposi's sarcoma. I was there with him when he died. I remember talking to a couple of very good friends the next morning. Brett had died in the middle of the night. And I said that it was right that he had died. He had suffered enough. And they said, "Oh, you feel that way now. You won't later." But I still say it was right.

When we found out that Michael had tested positive, it was like well, This can't be! This isn't possible. How are we going to do it?

So we struggled and worked to get through that. I really struggled to come to terms with death as a part of life. Sometimes I can't believe or understand *how* we're doing it. It's part of our life. *This* is our life. It doesn't do any good to feel sorry for ourselves. Doing that just makes it impossible to appreciate and enjoy what we do have.

Michael is on the holistic bent. Why? Well, he watched a brother die who had aggressively gone the other way. He has also had a more spiritual kind of bent. He lives in Santa Fe, New Mexico. So he won't take AZT. And one of the things we've really had to come to terms with, and respect, is that whatever Michael has to do for himself is the right thing for him to do.

Michael and I talk about the future a lot. He is out there living his life, and I want to support that; I don't want to think about his death. He's very determined he's going to beat this. He's trying alternative therapies and is actually having test results that are as-tonishing. It's scary. It's scary for all of us—*to believe*, you know? I'm walking a fine line of wanting to be hopeful, saying, "Yes, he's going to find a way to beat it." After all, if somebody is going to beat it, why shouldn't it be my son? And on the other side of this fine line is, Well, this is supposed to be a terminal disease.

What gets me through this?

I've become enormously spiritual. I really do believe that there is some sort of power energy force, and I don't know exactly what it is. And I believe that everyone finds it in their own way. It may be a Christ figure for one person, or a traditional image of God for someone else, or maybe a force of nature for someone else. I don't know. But I try, honestly, *to know*. I think one of my biggest goals is to try to really accept that I cannot control everything. All I can do is the best that I can do. And I hope to really keep growing, and by that I mean to keep opening my heart. I hope that it can continue to open. And through that, I hope to be able to help others. I also do a lot of volunteer work, which is very helpful to me.

What do I see when I look into the mirror?

Someone who has aged very rapidly.

What would I say to other mothers?

Just be there. Don't deny yourself or your son what *being there* means. Talk to other mothers and other people who have been through it. Reach out. Get support. Tell your friends, so that you can get their support. People who might react negatively I don't want around, anyway. I've even told people at work, and that was not easy. I mean it when I say, if they can't accept it, I don't want them as a part of my life.

You know, a lot of mothers, a lot of parents, have the whole issue of homosexuality to deal with as well. I remember we had thought, secretly, that each of the boys was gay before they came out or were open about it. And yet when they told us, it was still like "Whuuuppp!" You know, there *it* was. And I started feeling sorry for myself, thinking that I'm not going to be a grandmother, stuff like that. And then one day I woke up and just said to myself, What are you doing? They are exactly the same people they were before they told you this. Cut this *nonsense* out! Just accept it. It doesn't change your child or the person they are.

I would also tell them about the first meeting I went to with a group called MAP, Mothers of AIDS Patients. The thing that struck me the most in that meeting was that there were mothers there who had lost sons to AIDS and there they were, *functioning*. And I said to myself, They made it through, you'll make it through. You're a strong person. You'll make it through. And you know what? You do make it through.

The other thing is give in to the moment. Maybe that's what I was trying to say by "being there." Laugh. Cry. Go with whatever, wherever you're at. Because it's the only way you are going to get through. You don't have to be perfect. You don't have to be a hero.

—*BRENDA FREIBERG*

Jason Jasnos found out that he was HIV-positive in January 1989. He was 18 years old.

The man I was in a relationship with started getting sick. When we came back from a trip to Turkey, we put him into the hospital, after he had been telling me for weeks that he had salmonella. Eventually he got so sick that he couldn't hide it anymore, and he told me the truth. He also told me that I was HIV-positive. I had given blood at school, and they sent a certified letter to my mother that he had found and ripped up. He died a short time after.

When I found out I was HIV-positive, I immediately indulged in heavy alcohol and drugs. A "friend" of mine came over and introduced me to crack. I started smoking crack every day for about four months. Finally my mom had a clue that something was going on. I mean, I had lost 40 pounds and wasn't sleeping or eating. One morning I was coming down off crack and my body went into shock. I thought it was a symptom of AIDS. I freaked out. I went to my mom and told her that I was addicted to crack and needed help. I didn't tell her that I was HIV-positive. Finally she got around to prying, and when she got me to let her talk to my doctor, she found out everything.

I thought I was going to die every waking moment. I'd go to sleep and that was my reprieve. Then when I'd wake up, the first thing I thought was, Oh, shit. I'm going to die. What am I going to do? I thought, Why *me?* I'm so young, and this is not something that should be happening to me. I still have my whole life ahead of me, but it's going to end real soon.

After my mom found out about my addiction, I went and got treatment, and I've been clean and sober ever since. When I was first diagnosed, I said to myself that I was going to start exercising and all that, but I just didn't have the life force. I was very alone and felt very tired and weak. While I was in treatment, I gained a pound a day and got stronger. And while in treatment I met a 26-year-old girl and accidentally got her pregnant. Before we had sex, I told her that I was positive. This is a hard subject for me to talk about, but she had the baby. The baby is OK, and so is she. I thank God for that.

I pray for God's will for me. If it's my time to go, then it's my time to go. I won't argue with the way things are supposed to happen. Everything else is kind of obsolete. Whatever He wants, whatever is in my path that I need to accomplish, I pray for the strength to do it. Each little goal that I accomplish is something that gives me a spirit to want to live. I try not to get resentful. Resentment will kill me. If I feel anger, I have to let it out before it eats me up.

Today I'm in college studying art, art history, and interpersonal communications. I'm also doing part-time work and a lot of volunteer work, educating teens so that they won't ever get this virus. I've spoken in several schools, and each time it's amazing. I get up there and I'm totally terrified because I'm sharing all this personal stuff. I tell them and they listen, and they're really attentive, and they're shocked. I walk up there and I have a big build and am rather strong. I appear to be healthy and at the peak of my adolescence. So when I get up there, the last thing they expect me to say is that I'm HIV-positive.

I wish that I could have children and have a normal sex life. But when I look into the mirror, like when I'm brushing my hair, I say to myself, I hope I can love a lot of people today. I have a lot of love to give, and that's who I am today. As for tomorrow, I'd like to be with my son. I'd like to help raise him. I want to be a part of his life. For now, though, I just want to work on myself. I want to get so secure that I can be helpful in his life. So I'm doing the groundwork and setting the foundation for my life. That way, I can one day be a part of his.

—JASON JASNOS

☐ As of this writing, Jason Jasnos is still healthy, and still standing before teenagers as a mirror, a warning, an inspiration.

It was part of a routine physical with a new doctor. I really just wanted to rule out why I had had swollen lymph nodes for four years. So I got tested and didn't really think about it. And then I went back to the doctor for a B-12 shot, and he called me into his office. He said I had ARC, but he also said that I was really healthy and that I could remain healthy. Still, I instantly went into shock. I was numb.

My mom pressured me into going to two of the top specialists in Los Angeles. They were putting a lot of pressure on me to go on AZT, even though my T-cells were still really high. But I was into the natural, holistic path, so I argued with these doctors and never went back. I've been doing Chinese herbs and getting acupuncture for two years. I also started exercising a lot, and that's had a big impact on my life. I feel a lot better, mentally and physically.

The boyfriend that I had at the time freaked out. He thought he might have it, that I might have given it to him. We had been living together for a year. He was tested and it was negative, but for the next six months he was still freaking out. We stayed together for two more years, but it was totally platonic. He just totally physically withdrew from me. He wouldn't use the same bar of soap or the same towels. I felt like a leper. I thought that I had no options. That's why I stayed in that relationship, and it was really damaging to my self-esteem. The best thing was having him leave, getting out of that relationship.

I've been physically healthy, so the hardest thing for me has been the rejection that comes with relationships. It's really difficult to date a guy, to like a guy, and then get stressed out about telling him. That's happened before. There have been a couple of guys who just freaked out after I told them. My last boyfriend accepted it, but still he'd get anxious about it every so often. But there is hope. I've seen an HIV-positive, heterosexual woman and an HIV-negative man continue their relationship and get married. I know other HIV-positive couples who have gotten married.

What would I say to other women?

Women have been excluded from a lot of medical trials that have been designed just for men. Also, physical symptoms that women manifest having AIDS or being HIV-positive have been excluded from the criteria of what is officially considered AIDS, and so women have been unable to get insurance or disability.

I think one of the most important things, especially in the beginning, is to get involved in some kind of support group. I know that's what really helped me when I first found out, being with other HIV-positive people I could relate to. I think your emotional state plays a very big part in your physical state.

Also, do your own research. Don't just put all of your eggs in the basket of a traditional Western doctor.

This isn't a death sentence. You can live a long, happy, and fulfilled life being HIV-positive. And be *rebellious.* I think that's one of the main things that has kept me healthy. I'm rebellious and will not, and do not, accept the AIDS-equals-death mentality.

—ANDREA SKOPP

☐ Andrea Skopp was 24 years old when she was diagnosed with ARC in 1987. As of this writing she is still relatively healthy, working with adolescents in a mental-health facility, and speaking out about women and HIV.

We are all right here in the midst of everybody.

It became clear to me that I have a responsibility to other people with AIDS and HIV to not make it look like I'm frightened or ashamed or that I'm going to be intimidated by the consequences of being open about this disease. And ultimately, keeping it to myself somehow suggests that. If it doesn't come out until you're dying or dead, that's what people are left with.

> ☐ On November 25, 1991, Los Angeles Municipal Court
> Judge Rand Schrader, 46, held a press conference in his
> chambers announcing that he had AIDS. Judge Schrader
> had been diagnosed with pneumocystis and AIDS a
> month before. He had tested HIV-positive in 1989.
> Several months after he made his announcement, Judge
> Schrader consented to an interview for this book in
> which he reflected on his disease and on his decision to
> go public.

I've always been very public about being gay, and so that was already out there; I never had concern about that. But after I had pneumocystis, I felt that hiding it would be very difficult because I'm kind of well-known and it's hard to stop people from talking. It would have put me in the situation of constantly having to deny it.

210

It would have been a constant fabrication when someone asks, "How are you?" if you are not able to say, "Well, by the way, I was in the hospital and I've been pretty sick." I just didn't want to live my life that way. I didn't want to have to feel that I couldn't talk about this. There's really no reason *not* to talk about it. It's a fact.

In terms of people knowing, people have just been very nice, very caring. They reach out more and express their kindness and friendship more. Those things are the good that have come from this disease. I mean, there are real tremendous, positive effects when people learn this about you. You've given them a chance to tell you all the things they want to tell you. If you don't let them know you're sick, they can't tell you those things.

How has this affected my job?

In terms of what I handle in criminal law, I don't think I've changed, because you just follow the law. The law is the law, and that is pretty much the same. But I think I do try to be kinder, a little more understanding to people in my interactions with them.

What has gotten me through this?

I have always been a pretty positive person. It's crazy, but I'm not sad. There are times of feeling sadness, sure, but basically I enjoy my life. I guess my philosophy is a common one now, which is to enjoy what I have now and don't start mourning my loss of life before it's happened.

I do miss the mindlessness of feeling there's time. You miss the ambition that you had for the future. You miss a certain sexuality that you can't really practice, because you're going to have to be mindful of not infecting others. You also can't expose yourself to what others might give to you that your body can't handle anymore. These are losses that are sometimes hard for people who have AIDS to talk about. I'm not saying you can't be sexual, but I am saying you can't be as free.

211

What was my childhood ambition?

My childhood ambition was to be president of the United States. But I've since realized that no Jews have ever been elected president, so that probably would not have worked out anyway.

—JUDGE RAND SCHRADER

☐ As of this writing Judge Schrader is still relatively healthy and still sitting on the Los Angeles Municipal Court bench. He is the first and only known person with AIDS to sit and serve on the California bench.

John Robert Toves and Liza Joseph were an unlikely pair.
He was gay, she was straight. He was 32, she was 19.
And yet, they became the best of friends. As Liza
described their union, "Sometimes you meet someone
and everything falls into place. You don't have to try to
create a friendship. It just happens. If you're lucky, it
happens once in a lifetime. I've had my once in a
lifetime."

On Christmas of 1988 John was diagnosed with
Kaposi's sarcoma and AIDS. For the next year and a half
Liza remained a whisper away from John's side, their
bond growing deeper. Such was not the case with Brian,
their mutual good friend ("We were like the three
musketeers"), who moved back to his hometown of
Seattle.

On the day of John's death, March 10, 1990, Liza wrote
a letter to Brian detailing the last days and moments in
the life of the friend they shared. She has graciously
allowed us to reprint it below.

On Saturday morning, March 10, 1990, at 8:20, our John took his
last breaths in this world. I want to tell you everything because I
know that though you weren't there physically, you were with us.

From Thursday night till today, here is how John became free and how we suffered a loss which can only be compared to losing one of our own. John was, is, and always will be a part of our hearts.

When I arrived at the hospice on Thursday, I was so scared because John had started doing something which is called chain-stoking. It's a change in breathing people go through before they die. He was unconscious, which was something I had come to deal with in the previous couple of weeks. He seemed to be sleeping but would only rouse with a lot of effort from me. Almost as soon as I walked in there, I had to run out because he would only take about four breaths and then stop for about 20 seconds. I got one of the CNAs [certified nursing assistants] to look at him, and he confirmed what I already knew. It was getting close.

When I calmed down, I went back in and started to talk to him. "Johnnie, Johnnie, how are you?" "The other kind of fine," he said. "The other kind of fine? What other kind of fine?" I asked. "Does that mean it's time to go?" "Yes," he answered. Brian, my heart started to break. It wasn't as though it was any surprise to me, but *it* was really going to happen. I told him I was going to make him a milkshake, and he sat up and told me he was coming with me. Brian, he hadn't walked for nearly two weeks! He kept insisting that he was going to come, until he finally passed out again. When I came back with it, he took a tiny sip, but he couldn't swallow! He started choking, and although he was OK, that was the final loss for him. He had already lost most of his eyesight except for an occasional flash of clarity, he was mostly deaf, and he was completely incontinent and in diapers. This was not John. Anyway, not our strong, invincible John with all the answers. The next time he became lucid, he said what were to be the last words I ever heard from him. I was sitting on the bed by his side, alternately singing

214

to him and talking to him, crying all the while, and he opened his eyes and said, "You look so beautiful!" He spoke with absolute clarity, completely unlike his conversation of the past month, which was almost unintelligible. After that he lapsed back into unconsciousness, and the only reason I know that he could hear me as I sang and talked was because I never let go of his hand, and we would alternately squeeze each other as I went on. I decided, with the encouragement of the staff there [at the hospice], that it would be wise for me to stay because his time was so close, and the rest of my time that night was spent reassuring him that it was OK to let go, because I was there and I loved him. I sang him every song in my limited repertoire. I slept on a cot in his room, waking intermittently to hear the conversation of the nurses as they discussed his breathing, which eventually stabilized, which is not to say that it was normal, only *more* normal.

As I had only had about four hours of sleep, I had to go home after work before I went back to be with him once again. I guess I knew what was about to happen, because I had a few drinks, a pot of coffee, and a shower before I felt ready to face the situation again.

When I got back, there was something different about him. Not only could I not wake him for love or money, but after about an hour he wouldn't squeeze my hand. His little hands started to grow cold. One of the CNAs, Triva, came in with me and confirmed my suspicions that it was time. She told me not to stay in the room all the time because sometimes people wouldn't let go when the ones they loved were there. . . . It was at 6:30 the next morning when I woke up with Triva there telling me that John's breathing was so bad that she thought I should be by his side. All the time I was by his side, I kept rewinding "The Rose" and singing it over and over again. . . . I went to pick up his hand. It was all curled up in a fist, and when I unclenched it, I pulled back because it was freezing cold . . . and blue. Then I noticed his face, which, though already painfully thin, had turned white and his KS was black. I ran down and got Triva, Karen, and Rick [the CNAs] and begged them to come up, which they did, and immediately Rick went to get oxygen. They held me and told me it was nearly over.

They hooked up the oxygen. . . . [Then] I screamed because our Johnnie stopped breathing. Karen took me out of the room for a minute because they hooked him up again and he started to breathe. I begged Rick to "put 'our song' on!" As it played and as I stood in the arms of three people whom I couldn't have been without, John Robert Toves, a friend to whom I owe so much, who touched everyone with whom he came in contact, who never received the blessings in this life which he had earned, was finally at peace. It was 8:20 A.M.

Brian, after that it was a matter of going back in and saying good-bye to John's spirit, which was finally free. I looked out at the sun and the sky—it was such a beautiful day—and I told Johnnie everything that was in my heart. He will never leave us as long as we remember the blessings of love and wisdom which were his gifts to us. Gifts he was always ready to give. Gifts he all too seldom received.

He is being cremated, and his ashes will be scattered at sea, once more giving any earthbound parts of his spirit the freedom to fly at last to the heaven he deserves more than anyone I've ever known.

—*LIZA JOSEPH*

I want to describe to you what it feels like to find out that you are HIV-positive. A couple of weeks ago, my mother asked me, "How do you feel?" And I said, "Well, Mom, the only way I can describe it to you is like this: You know the feeling you get when you've gotten off the bus and you realize that you've left your wallet on the seat, and the bus is taking off? You realize that it's *that* close to you, but the bus is taking off and you'll never see it again. That's how I feel being HIV-positive. My life is never, ever going to be the same again. The bus has taken off."

The night Chris and I found out that we were HIV-positive was three months after the San Francisco earthquake. I had lost my apartment and was kind of thrown into this situation where I was living with Chris. I used his razor and his toothbrush. Shortly after, he went to the dentist for some minor surgery. It took about a month and a half for his mouth to heal. Every time he kissed me, I would taste blood, and I thought, "Hey, there's something wrong here." That's when he said, "Well, I'd better go get tested." He had told me before that he was HIV-negative. I had been tested before and was also HIV-negative. Anyway, he was afraid to go alone and he said, "If I go, will you go with me?" And I said, "Sure, I'll go with you. It's no big deal." So I went with him. We got tested two weeks before we moved into our new apartment. We were moving in together for the first time. Then, on January 10, 1990, we went to get

217

our results. We had spent the whole day moving. And then, at 7:00 P.M., we were both told that we were positive.

Needless to say, that night was crazy. We couldn't sleep. I had that feeling in my stomach, like the world was going to end. It didn't go away for weeks and weeks. Going through it, you wonder if it will ever go away, but it does. You get used to the idea of it, and in time, you begin to think of other things again.

I didn't want to lie back and let whatever happened happen. I aggressively researched clinical trials and decided to volunteer for the Salk HIV-immunotherapy, which I've now been involved with for a year and a half. I've spent a lot of money to be a part of it. I fly to Los Angeles from San Francisco once, sometimes twice a month. In the course of the study my T-cells dropped considerably at a stressful point in 1991, and I was put on AZT, 500 milligrams a day. The trials have been very hush-hush. I'm in a double-blind placebo control trial. I understand that there are 10 volunteers in several major cities, and I'm one of 10 in the Los Angeles study. Five of us have been given placebo. I would expect that I have been given placebo, considering that my T-cells dropped as much as they did in August. They dropped 400 points in a matter of a month and a half. Why did I want to participate in the study? I wanted to do my part in finding a cure. I wanted to be a voice of hope in my own way. There was so much badness happening all around me.

I've seen two very important men in my life, both good friends and good lovers, progress in the disease from being vital, healthy men to their deaths. How do you describe that? Dennis was very ill. He had KS lesions all over his body. When we would go out to the grocery store, people would stare and point. We'd be in the produce section and people would run out. Then he had to get out of his apartment. At that point he hadn't gotten so bad that he couldn't go to the bathroom. He was still able to walk and cook a

218

little bit. So I said to him, "You just come stay with me." And so we planned on him moving in after Christmas. Then, about a week into December, Chris went to the doctor because he had been getting thinner and was having these terrible pains in his stomach and throat. He was diagnosed with throat cancer. After having to deal with this virus for a year with Dennis, I just fell apart. I had gotten to a point where I just didn't think that I would be able to watch my friends get sicker and sicker. The thought of Chris having KS in his throat and having to go through chemotherapy and radiation was just too much. I really felt suicidal at that time. I just didn't want to watch my friends die.

That day I went to church, and the sermon was dealing with the losses of our friends and how to get through it. In a nutshell, the preacher said that all you can do is do everything you can for your friends, know in your heart that you did everything you could, and not be complacent and complain and watch the world fall apart around you. Even though that's what I was doing all along, I hadn't had anybody actually say those words to me. Life didn't become great at that point, but it became bearable.

People warned me that I was jeopardizing my own health by taking care of them, because my own T-cells were dropping. But I couldn't see any other way than to be with them every minute that I could, as long as I could. I'm really glad that I did. I had some of the most precious, personal moments with these men just days before they died. My lover Dennis died in April of 1991. And then my lover Chris died in October of 1991. It was a pretty horrible year.

What gets me through this?

I still talk to Dennis and Chris a lot. I feel like I have guardian angels. I miss them so much, and I feel their presence very strongly. I mean, weird things have happened in this house that people just don't believe. Things have actually moved in front of my face. There was about a week and a half where it was happening every day. It's a comforting thought. It's something that's helped me get on with my life. After Chris died, I couldn't even pull myself out of bed. I just wanted to sleep the rest of my life away. Then, when these things began happening in the house a few weeks later, I felt like I wasn't alone anymore. Somehow I felt good again. I started going back to school. I'm even sort of optimistic about the future. I think if I've got five years of healthy time left, I think it's possible that there might be a cure. If there isn't, then I'm just going to take these classes that I've always wanted to take and just shoot for graduation—make my mother happy.

What do I see when I look in the mirror?

I just kind of see an unsure face looking back. The future is so uncertain. You can't count on anything. I could be sick next year. When I look in the mirror I see concern. Not so much for my own mortality anymore, because if that happens, it happens. I'm not afraid of death anymore. I've seen it. It's been here in this house with me. I fear how it could affect my family. I wouldn't want them to go through what I've seen.

What do I miss most?

That I can't bench press 175 pounds anymore. Seriously, my childhood ambition was to have 10 children. I always thought I would have my first by the time I was 25, and here I am, 33 and HIV-positive. All I ever wanted to be was a father, and that's what broke my heart the most that day in January, when I realized that that day would never be.   *—RIAN NEVES*

☐ As of this writing Rian Neves is still living in San Francisco and still going to school, studying filmmaking. He has completed a student film about the life and death of his lover, Chris.

    Chris Wall died of AIDS at the age of 31; Dennis Tate died at the age of 29.

Shirley Androlewicz's 37-year-old son, Michael, was diagnosed with AIDS on April 6, 1987. At first, in an effort to retain his independence, Michael resisted returning to his parents' home—until he no longer could. And then he learned what having a family is all about.

Michael came home for Christmas, and I *knew* then. I knew before he did. Maybe he knew but didn't want to know. Then, in April, he was hospitalized. The minute I walked into the AIDS ward, everything I knew was confirmed. Then, when the doctor came into the room, he asked Michael if he wanted him to tell me everything. Michael said, "Yes, tell her." He had pneumocystis and AIDS. Michael closed his eyes and didn't open them for a long time. Finally he said, "I'm so sorry, Mom." I said, "Don't be sorry. Let's see what we can do about it."

Michael had an apartment in Los Angeles. When he'd feel good, he'd come home to San Diego and would be fine, and all of sudden you'd just watch him go downhill. I'd run back and forth to and from L.A. because he didn't want to give up his apartment. He didn't want to give up, you know? It got to be hard on me running back and forth all the time. The train ride was about three hours.

He asked us to please not tell any of our friends. The social worker at the hospital said, "You'll find that it's not very accepted and you'll lose a lot of friends." So we didn't tell anybody. That was hard. I would never do that again. I would say to people, "If you don't like me or if you don't like my son, *I don't care!*"

Michael always had a way of trying to hide things from us. To give you a hint, his father was the chief of police, very polished and hard-nosed. They had a great respect for each other and a great love for each other, but Michael was afraid to tell his father anything. He was afraid that he wouldn't approve. As for Michael's younger brother, Steven, Michael carried a letter around with him that I found after he died. It was from Steven and it said, "I love you very much. You're my brother. Whatever your sexual persuasion is, that's your business. We love you because you're you. Don't stay away from us for that reason."

When Michael finally came home to live and everyone in the family knew he had AIDS, it was a relief. It was just like the weight of the world was off our shoulders. By then Michael had CMV-retinitis and had gone blind. That was the hardest part. I got a baby monitor and put it in his room so that I could hear him. He hallucinated, and I could hear him move in the bed, so I didn't get any sleep. It was every two hours or so that he would walk into a wall or just fall, so it got to a point where I just slept on the floor beside his bed.

I got him up every morning and made him eat, gave him his medicine, and put him in a hot tub of water. I said to him, "I'm your mother and I've seen everything you've got. It's nothing to me. So please don't think of me in that way." That was very embarrassing for him to deal with, but after a while he just got used to it. I kept him spotlessly clean. That's so important. Michael never got an infection while he was home. He got them in the hospital, but never at home.

My husband was the most loving thing with Michael. He'd get up in the middle of the night to take care of him and never said anything about it. Michael's friends came into our house, which was a very difficult thing for my husband to accept. He had never seen guys kiss and put their arms around each other.

Michael was home for six and a half months before he died. He wanted to be cremated. Today he sits up on my hearth. I have him in my egg collection, in a big egg, and nobody knows that he's there. I had asked him where he wanted his ashes to be buried, and he said that he didn't know. I asked him what should we do with them if we moved back to St. Louis. He said, "You'll have to take me with you." I told him, "I'll carry you around in my purse. We'll go to the movies together."

What would I say to other mothers?

Love that child. When he shakes, hold him. When he gets cold, wrap a blanket around him. Hold him. He likes that. It's so important that they know that they're not the "garbage" people said they were. They deserve every dignity in the world. They're human. When I was in that hospital, there were so many boys on that floor whom nobody visited. I thought, "How terrible; how could you do this to your child? How could you do that?"

—SHIRLEY ANDROLEWICZ

☐ Today, in her son Michael's name and memory, Shirley Androlewicz is a volunteer with Momma's Kitchen, an AIDS services group that prepares and delivers meals to homebound people with AIDS.

PEP (Peer Education Programs) is comprised of a group of teenagers who educate other teens about HIV and AIDS.

It is a group that Shellye Howard, now 18, turned to when she learned that her father was HIV-positive.

I was brought to PEP L.A. after my father was diagnosed HIV-positive. I felt that I wanted to take the anger I had and turn it into something positive. I felt the most positive thing I could do was get out there and educate other people about HIV and AIDS—not only about how it's contracted, but also about how the people who have contracted it are still human beings with feelings and emotions.

My dad is a hemophiliac, and that's how he got the disease. At the time, his doctors told him that there wasn't a lot to worry about, that very few people converted from HIV-positive to AIDS. At the time, in 1985, things were a little different in terms of AIDS and HIV than they are today. It wasn't considered to be something quite so scary. So it wasn't really something that was hard for him to tell us, it was just a part of an ordinary conversation. We really didn't think too much about it.

Once we got to a point that doctors realized we should be worrying, I thought, Oh my God, what will happen? Will he make it to my graduation?

I think for the first time I was forced to face the fact that human beings are mortal. It's made me more careful. I think twice about not only *who* I'm going out with, but *what* I'm doing when I am going out. When my father was diagnosed, I was in the seventh grade. So basically I was aware of the dangers before I hit the stage of wanting to experiment. So I'm not experimenting with sex. I'm not running around with a whole bunch of different guys every night of the week. I'm not experimenting with drugs. I'm staying far away from that.

It's also taught me to treat other human beings with compassion and respect, especially those who may be a little different from what America may consider the norm. These people are still worth getting to know. They are still good human beings, even if there is a virus running around in their body.

I feel that I have the potential to make a difference in other people's lives. I know I make more of a difference talking to teens about sex education, abstinence, proper condom use, and safer sex than a 60-year-old man would. When an adult shares the information, unfortunately, most of the time it's ignored. But, when a teen shares the information, other teens listen; it brings the issue home; we understand each other.

What would I say to other teens?

The first thing I'd say is, "Wake up." A lot of teens think that they're immortal. We need to know that AIDS does not discriminate against anyone. And because of that, now is not the time to experiment with sex or drugs. Through experimentation, you can end up catching a disease that there is no cure for. It's not worth it for one hit, and it's not worth it for one night of sex with a boyfriend or girlfriend. It's just not worth it. Your life is more important.

What was my childhood ambition?

My dream ever since I was a little girl was to be a famous actress. What I've found out, though, is that I really enjoy working with people. If I can make their lives a little easier, it's far more satisfying than going up on the stage and delivering a monologue or singing a song.

—SHELLYE HOWARD

□ As of this writing Shellye Howard is a freshman in college, majoring in psychology.

Shellye's father tested HIV-positive in 1985 at the age of 37. As of this writing he is still relatively healthy. Says Shellye, "When I look into the future and think about the family and children that I might have when I get older, I wonder, Will Dad be there to share those times with me?"

*H*ow do I begin? I started caring less about things—about other people's things. I focused more on myself. I've become real selfish in a way. I really don't want to hear about other people's problems, because I've got my own to deal with.

I feel like I've let other people down. It's like my grandma and I were really close. She's 84 years old. Naturally, I always planned on her going long before me. Now there's a distinct possibility that my grandma might see me put in the ground, and that tears me to pieces. That's the worst part of this whole thing for me.

This has brought my family closer together; it's affected my whole family. It took me four months of going to see a psychologist before I could tell my parents that I was HIV-positive. We weren't real close, although my dad's always been real close with my brothers. When your family has not been real close, all of a sudden something like this happens and they want to be your best friend, but you don't know how to handle them as your best friend. My sister has done volunteer work for Project Ahead [an AIDS services organization in Long Beach, California]. And my dad and I are basically closer than we've ever been. But every time he sees me, he says, "Well, you're looking good today." And the past three times he's said that, I had been really sick. That's very frustrating. It's like he wants to believe that I'm better, or whatever. But even though he is having a real hard time accepting it, he's very aware.

My mom and I have worked intensely on our relationship. We're closer than we have ever been. Only my mother knows or has accepted how serious this is. My brothers, sisters, grandmother, and dad have not. That makes it real hard.

It's difficult being labeled as "infected." I'm single, and it's very hard. I date, but I play safe. I won't let anyone touch me.

What do I see when I look in the mirror?

Kind of like, hopelessness. I'm sorry, but it's been one of those weeks. I've lost too many friends. One of my friends was as healthy as can be. We went to lunch the day before he died. He went to sleep that night and just had a stroke [AIDS-related] and died!

What gets me through this?

I believe in the Master Plan. When it's my turn to go, it means that my mission here is finished.

I was fortunate enough to fly to Kansas City for Christmas. I have a cousin there will full-blown AIDS. I hadn't seen him in 20 years. It was very comforting, and we developed a wonderful bond. He was a great inspiration to me.

I have so much more that I want to do. I have so many more things that I want to see. I went to the Grand Canyon when I was six years old, but I don't remember it. And I want to see Yellowstone Park. And the redwood forest. And . . .

—TODD WRIGHT

☐ Todd Wright was diagnosed with ARC on April 29, 1991. He is 28 years old.

This disease is a blessing in disguise, and I'm starting to feel that more and more. I feel like it's a wake-up call from God. A year and a half ago I went through one of the biggest changes that this disease has brought into my life: my recovery from addiction to alcohol. I think I would have drunk myself to death if not for this disease.

This last year and a half has just been marvelous. I've been sick on and off, but my whole attitude has changed. I'm going on seven years now. I tested HIV-positive in 1985. I'm one of the long-term survivors. I've educated myself about my disease, and I take part in my treatment. I also have a positive attitude. I've gotten back to spiritual things, I'm into meditation, and I've gone back to college. I'm taking a chemical-dependency course at Mission College. I'd like to be a counselor in chemical dependency.

I have a son who's 24 and a daughter who's 30. I don't believe they've been tested. I've been urging them to do it, but they won't. I think they're afraid, and I think they're in denial about Mom. My daughter knows more about the disease, and she's more attentive concerning it, but my son just seems to brush it off. Still, I have a better relationship now with my children, family, and friends.

What do I see when I look in the mirror?

Today I see kind of a scruffy-looking lady. Usually, in the morning, one of my exercises is to look in the mirror, right into my own eyes, and tell myself how much I love and approve of myself. I give myself strokes.

What do I miss most?

Absolutely nothing. I do more now than I did then.

What are my future goals?

Well, I'm 50 years old and I'm a slow learner. It took me to age 48 to start learning. I still smoke, and I don't exercise enough. It's interesting that you asked about goals. I was reading a book and it said to start out with 10, you know, small ones. I've never been a goal maker, but I want to continue with school and with my commitment to health and exercise. And, oh, a third one: a man in my life. I would like that to be a goal. I miss that!

—JOAN LEE

☐ Joan Lee, now 51, was diagnosed with ARC in the beginning of 1990. As of this writing she is still relatively healthy and still pursuing her goals—all three of them.

William Bonney was David Lindsey's friend, former lover, and former business partner when he was diagnosed with AIDS. David and his new boyfriend, Randy West, invited Williams to live in their home, where they took care of him until his death.

I was at a crucial point in my life. Bill and I had just lost a business. It was the first time I had ever really failed at something. I kind of went off the deep end and our relationship changed. I went my way and got involved with Randy, and he went his. Then Bill got sick, and one of the best things Randy could have done for me was to say, "Bring him down here, and we'll take care of him."

Bill just had a very wonderful outlook on life. He would see other people who were going through it, and he would take great heart in the fact that he wasn't alone. He was never the type of person who sat there and said, "Why me?" He was marvelous inspiration.

Anyway, we moved him into the front upstairs bedroom. This was toward the last six months of his life. He was on liquid morphine, and he would just rest all day. Even though our relationship had changed, there was still an incredible love there. We basically clung to each other in many respects. I had had many other friends die, but this was different. This was my lover dying.

There was one thing that Bill looked forward to every day. I'd go upstairs and he'd say, "How many more hours? How many hours until—Vanna White?" And I'd say, "Well, it's about four o'clock, so three hours." And he'd go, "Yeah!" He loved to see her different clothes, and he used to predict what she was going to wear. She was just beginning her meteoric rise at that time.

We had a very large living room with virtually no furniture in it, except for this tiny little loveseat that sat right in front of a 45-inch television set. Bill was very, very unsteady on his feet at that time. He had really wasted away to skin and bones. I would go in and pick him out of his bed and carry him into the living room and put him on the loveseat. And Randy would come in, and they would sit there and laugh. I took great comfort in knowing that Randy felt like he was doing something for Bill. He'd make him laugh. Then they'd sit there, and for half an hour they'd watch Vanna White. That was the highlight of Bill's day. As soon as the show was over, he was ready to go back to bed. We'd pick him up, take him to bed, tuck him in, and he would generally fall asleep.

After Bill passed away, Randy and I tested, and we both found out that we were HIV-positive. What I'm now going through with Randy is an entirely different ball of wax from what I went through with Bill. They're two entirely different people; one who kind of accepted what he was going through and made the best of it, and one who is very, very angry about it.

What has gotten me through Bill's death?

I take great comfort in knowing that I made him happy and that he was as comfortable as he could be. I think I certainly had many wonderful friends to bury my grief in. I didn't go to any support groups; I just kept myself very busy and preoccupied my mind with work.

What would I say to other people?

Our happiness here on a daily basis is the most important thing. I don't plan a retirement. I have a very wonderful 16-year-old daughter who knows everything. When she and I are together, we enjoy every day to the fullest. I'm not waiting for her to graduate so I can take her skiing in Switzerland. What I am able to do for her now, I do *now*.

—*DAVID LINDSEY*

☐ William Bonney died on June 17, 1984, after suffering from six bouts of pneumocystis followed by cryptococcal meningitis. He was 42 years old.

As of this writing, David Lindsey and Randy West are still together and still relatively healthy. They are also in business together with the greeting-card company, West Graphics.

Freddie Weber is a singer/actress/songwriter who for the past three years has been feeding nourishment, both food and spiritual, to people with AIDS. Freddie operates Project Angel Food, an AIDS service organization that delivers meals to homebound people with AIDS.

As an actress and a writer I used to just sort of sit around and wait for the phone to ring. So one day I just got on my knees and said to God, "Use me."

I was a volunteer for Louise Hay, and then I worked with the Los Angeles Center for Living. I did everything, anything. What happened to me with people with AIDS, being around people with AIDS, was that they weren't like other people I knew. They seemed so naked. It was like somebody had opened their hearts. It was like they had no defenses like there are with most people. They would be so loving, it just made my heart open up. I just fell in love, and it was like a God shot, like God zapping me, you know? This is *it* for you. You're in love. *Go!* So I did a lot of volunteer work, and then Marianne Williamson [of the Los Angeles Center for Living], who knows these kinds of things, just looked at me and said, "I want you to start Project Angel Food. There are people who are homebound who need food delivered. So start it!"

I didn't have a clue about *how* to do it. I didn't know anything, which turned out to be the best thing, because God chose like an empty vessel, someone who would totally surrender to it. So I just did everything that channeled through me. And now we've got it all, in a weird kind of way. I mean, our filing system is weird, everything is by first names and is organized with yellow stickies. But it gets done. Two hundred sixty meals a day are served, and they are served with love.

We see a lot of people die, we work with death all the time, but you see the people come together here for this wonderful, amazing purpose, and we feel like we're a part of God, like little angels. It's that buoyant kind of love feeling that gets us through every day. We cry. Our hearts have been totally broken, and that's OK. We just love, cry, laugh, fall down and giggle, and make food. And when we deliver it, we just make jokes to the guys and hug them and cry. And we see them die, and we see them *live*.

What do I say to clients?

First I just listen. And I pray before I go in because I don't know what to do, what to say, and I still don't. I don't have any preconceived stuff in my head about what to do or say. So I pray and I ask God to guide me. And I may go in and make jokes, or I may go in and be insulting. I told one guy, "You're so *weird!*" and he just laughed. But mostly I listen. They want to talk. They want to talk so badly. And I hug them, and I feed them, and I love them.

I'm willing to fall in love over and over.

—FREDDIE WEBER

☐ Today, Freddie Weber continues to spread her messages of love and light, and both are contained in the brown paper packages that are delivered daily to homes all over Los Angeles. She has also written a song for and about people with AIDS that she has allowed us to reprint on the following page.

235

HEROES

By Freddie Weber

Men and women everywhere
leaving in the night
Don't know why and don't
know where,
Fading out of sight
Going towards the light

Heroes, my heroes
Fighting such a fight
Heroes, my heroes
of the night, of the night

Heroes, where are my heroes
Where do they go?
Where do they fly?
Are you a star in the
sky shining bright?

You came to earth, to
do a special mission
You volunteered,
it was your own decision
You went thru fire and
pain, gave up your armor,
lost damn everything
except your honor

Stand naked and alone,
your hearts are open
We're so shaken and alone,
our hearts are broken
How we cry
Oh God, how we cry
at night when you die

Angels, you are my angels
Sent down from God above
Your burning flame,
taught us all how to love

Heroes, heroes, beings
of the light
Heroes, my heroes
of the night.

I was diagnosed with AIDS on the very day they aired "An Early Frost" on television. If I had not watched that film, I actually don't think that I could have picked up my toys and gotten out of the sandbox and started dealing with the issue. The film got me out of denial that night.

I was a general contractor, and then the economy got shitty. So I decided to close the business. I now work as office manager for Tuesday's Child. It was time for me to give back to the community.

Now I live a more honest, truthful life. I don't put up with anybody's bullshit. I don't knowingly create madness and havoc in my life. I try to rid my life of all the stresses, even though being office manager of a foundation is full of stress—but it seems to be positive stress. I travel a lot. I treat myself well.

I took up skydiving after I was diagnosed. I've always lived life on the edge. I always will. I think that a lot of people, after they've been diagnosed, give up whatever their life is. They throw away the good parts of their life, and they don't address the bad parts. I've kept all of the good parts, and I realized that I had to address all the bad parts. I had to look at them, I had to own them, I had to forgive myself for them, and then I had to let them the f—k go. And then I could get on with my life and get on with my healing to whatever degree I was able to heal myself.

I'm allergic to all the antivirals. I have a violent reaction to every one of them. I'm just not willing to live my life that way.

What gets me through this?

Having been a bodybuilder and competitor, the gym is a very integral part of my life. It starts all of my days. It is what I love doing. It has kept me a fit person, and it has also helped me to mentally deal with this.

All of my peers are dead. I have lost over 40 people. My lover died of AIDS. Nobody I grew up with is alive today. Nobody but me. So it sounds very hard and cold, but it has become a matter of fact with me. Every time I hear that another friend of mine has passed away, it takes the wind out of me. I usually have to sit down, and a very strange feeling comes over me. But I don't cry anymore. Whether it is because of an illness or old age or AIDS, we're all going to pass. We are just not trained in my generation to talk about death, to accept death.

I have a very strange philosophy. I think AIDS in many ways was a gift to the planet. It has radically changed and moved a mass consciousness of a mass group of people. It has shaken them to the very core, and today it has made many of them better people for it. It seems that in history, if you look back, every time we get to a certain point in history, some major epidemic or major kind of health crisis hits the world to shake us to our very roots, to bring us back to some semblance of humanity. I think that AIDS has done this.

What would I say to others?

I learned a long time ago not to give advice, because, you know, advice and a dime won't get you a cup of coffee. What I would say is that each person needs to find out very quickly who they really are. I think they need to sit down and turn themselves inside out. Then, after they've done that, I think they need to find their metaphysical beliefs, whatever they may be, their power, their God, if you will. And I think they need to get in touch with that and ask for guidance. And they need to get honest with themselves. They need to stop living whatever lies they are living. And they need to accept the fact that they have been diagnosed with AIDS—and they are not an ugly person in any way, nor are they different from anyone else.

—BILL SEAN-HIX

☐ Bill Sean-Hix is 51 years old. He was diagnosed with cryptosporidiosis and AIDS in October 1985. As of this writing he is still working for the AIDS foundation and still relatively healthy.

I'm HIV-positive and I'm 16 years old. I thought that I could never get it because I was too cute. I broke up with the guy who gave it to me. He didn't even tell me that he had it. All my friends were telling me that he had the virus, so I went and got tested. My doctor didn't have the heart to tell me that I had the virus, so my therapist told me. I still went with the same guy for about a month, but I stopped having sex with him. Then he went to Hawaii for a week and I found somebody else. He is also HIV-positive, and he introduced me to crack. From that moment on I was addicted to crack. Now I'm struggling to stay sober.

I've had an alcohol problem since the age of 6. When I was 12, I got into drugs. From the ages of 5 to 11, I was molested by my mom's boyfriends. Also by their family members, neighborhood people, and kids at school—by anybody who knew I was easily taken advantage of. I went through a hell of a lot. When I was 11, my mom had remarried and I didn't like her husband, so I ran away to the streets of Hollywood. I've been in and out of juvenile hall, group homes, foster homes and one time I even went to the California Youth Authority. They called me "incorrigible."

Right now I'm in a runaway shelter called Options House. It's

a two-week program for teens who run away from home. So far I'm
the most street-experienced kid there. Some of the kids don't quite
understand a lot, and they're very judgmental, but I get along with
them pretty well. From here I'm going to go to a group home called
GLASS, Gay and Lesbian Adolescent Social Services. They accept
HIV-positive teens, but they have certain requirements that the teens
have to follow in order to stay there.

What do I see when I look in the mirror?

I see a teenager who knows what he wants; he just doesn't
know how to go about getting it. I want to better myself, get myself
off the streets. I want to be a counselor. Sometimes, though, I don't
have the motivation for it or the patience to keep going to school.
Basically, I hate school. The last grade I fully went through and
completed was the sixth grade. But my long-term goal is to become
a peer educator, and I know that I first have to go through school
and get an education.

When I look in the mirror, I also say, "You're a good person. I
love you. And you are *so* good-looking!" Sometimes it works.

What would I say to other teenagers?

That you aren't too cute, you aren't too rich, you aren't too
good, and you aren't too tough to get this disease. And I would say
to them that it is not the end of the world if they do get it. You don't
have to try and kill yourself. You won't die automatically. You will
live, and you can live for a long time and never get sick. And no
matter what happens, even if you come down with full-blown AIDS,
you are still a good person.

I preach safe sex. I don't preach that abstinence stuff. I think
that's just bull crap. I have talked to teenagers, and I say, "I know
you're going to have sex. So if you do, put on a condom. Just try it
out. And if you think you're too large, you're not. And if you think

you won't feel it, get a thinner condom. But use a condom and use it right."

What do I miss most?

Saying, "No, I'm negative."

—ALEX CHAMPION

☐ As of this writing Alex Champion has become active in public speaking, teaching other teenagers about AIDS. He has also found a stable home environment in which he hopes to remain until he turns 18. When he was asked his childhood ambition, Alex replied, "I wanted to be a police officer. And an actor. And a writer. And a singer. Now I just want to get my GED [graduation equivalency diploma]."

I tested HIV-positive in 1986. I am a recovering alcoholic and addict. When I went into treatment at the hospital, they gave me a bunch of blood tests, one of which happened to be an HIV test. I had no knowledge of the test, and this was before the laws came out protecting people from getting tested against their will.

The way I was told was very nonchalant. The doctor who gave me my post-test results acted like it didn't really matter that I was HIV-positive. He acted like I should decide whether or not I wanted to continue with the rehabilitation program, because I was going to die in a year anyway. I felt betrayed. I felt like this man was willfully telling me, You might as well *not* use the tools we've given you, and go out and kill yourself, drink yourself to death, drug yourself to death, because it's not going to matter anyway.

I was also numb. When you're given information that powerful, I think one goes into shock. And then, of course, there's denial. That couldn't be *me*. That's the first thing I thought, because I can remember in the early 1980s, in the community from which I came, the only people who were supposed to have this infection were gay white men. I certainly wasn't gay. And I certainly wasn't white. And I certainly wasn't a man!

I was scared to death about telling my husband. Would he abandon me? That's one of the first things I thought about. He was the only person in my life I could trust. And I just decided that whatever was gonna be was gonna have to be. He was shocked. But my husband knew a lot more about HIV than I did, which really made a difference. He held my hand and talked to me and told me that this didn't mean that I was going to have to die. The doctor had told me that I would be dead in a year. Who was I to believe? I was very confused.

I thought that God had betrayed me. God had abandoned me. I'm not a deeply religious person, but I was brought up to believe in a power greater than myself. And I just didn't consider myself a person worthy of getting something as cruel as this. I felt like a low animal. I took on all the ugly, nasty things that society was saying about people with HIV or AIDS. I took everything they projected and ran with it. That was my fault. I didn't have to accept that. I didn't have to believe that. I needed to have a greater understanding of who I was and what this virus actually was.

My husband had to get tested. He and I had had unprotected sex for over two years. I held my breath for about two weeks. Then, when his results came back, he said to me, "Listen. I know I'm negative." I held on to him for dear life. It was a very tight hold, a very tight hold.

I was diagnosed with AIDS and CMV-retinitis in July of 1991. I went into the hospital on my birthday, October 10, because I had a lot of pain in the back of my leg. On October 15, I couldn't walk. It's called polyreticulitis. It's when the nerves are separated from the strands, like when you have a nerve and the top of it comes off.

I walk a lot. Rather, I used to walk a lot. My job entailed a lot of walking. I'm a case manager and health educator, so I had to walk from one end of the campus to the other on a daily basis.

My husband, Mack, and I are very close. He's real funny, a comedian. He's taken it very hard, but it hasn't shown. He said the reason he feels a lot better about things is because of the way I've been handling it. I guess if I had broken down, he would've been a nervous wreck. When I went into the hospital the last time and my legs were affected by this disease, it was the first time I've ever seen him really stressed out. I told him, "You know, I'm going to be very honest with you. I'm going to fight like hell to walk." And I've done that. I'm doing pretty good. I'm very independent in the wheelchair now, and I do a lot of exercise. I am going to walk again. I plan on going back to work, and when I do, I hope to be walking with either a cane or a walker.

Why have I chosen to speak out about AIDS?

I believe if there had been someone visible in the early 1980s, I might not have this infection. I don't know when I contracted it, but I do know that the guy I was living with in 1983 died of a pulmonary infection or pneumonia. They didn't give the specific kind of pneumonia.

I don't believe that anyone should have to suffer with this illness. Before, I did not know what AIDS did to people. Then when I became involved in the [AIDS education] movement, I began to see my constituents die, and it broke my heart. They were being mistreated, punished, and ridiculed by a society that did not know what was going on. I had to watch them die a horrible death. And these were wonderful people. These people were not derelicts. They were not sinners. They were people who contracted a very ugly disease.

As a result I felt that this was too important not to share. I especially wanted women to know what I knew, because I began to see how many women around me were being impacted by this disease—professional women, women from the street, women who

246

have families. So I had to speak out. I really can't explain it, but I was compelled to do something, and this is what I chose to do.

You can't keep what you have unless you give it away.

What would I say to others?

Women are susceptible to getting HIV regardless if they use drugs or not. And I think we've got to stop doing that in the 1990s. I think labeling people as "these are the ones who will get this infection" has caused other people to feel that they have some kind of freedom. As a result there are more people getting infected.

I don't believe that others will be going through what I went through, and I'll tell you why. The scientific community has really come together in helping people to not develop symptoms so fast. I think there are people walking around now who have been infected for 10 years and they're not symptomatic. I have a girlfriend who's had it for seven years. She's not symptomatic at all, and her T-cell count is 750. And another thing is that people are not so ashamed and guilty that they're HIV-positive anymore. People like myself and Pedro Zamora are speaking out to show people the faces of AIDS and how we have managed to keep our heads held high. I don't think society is laying it on us so hard anymore. Slowly but surely it has ebbed its way into their lives too. I'm finding more and more people being compassionate to the cause as a result of their being personally affected. The first thing they say to me is, "Well, why didn't somebody tell me?" The fact is, somebody has been talking, but they weren't listening.

What would I say to others? Keep your heads high. Maintain a sense of pride and dignity at all costs. No one goes out and asks for AIDS or HIV. It's contracted out of ignorance, really. If we could get everybody to be responsible, then there would be no AIDS. That's the best thing I can say. That's the one thing that I've fought for: some self-respect and some dignity.

What do I see when I look in the mirror?

My eyes don't shine like they used to. My smile isn't as bright. But I'm still holding on. I'm still an attractive woman. Inside there's fear and a great deal of pain. The pain is that I won't be able to be with someone I really love. I really love my husband and my mom. I fear that I won't have that much time with them.

There's one more thing I'd like to say:

I'm not the enemy. The AIDS virus is the enemy. AIDS itself is the enemy. It just so happens that I am living with this disease. I work my butt off to make sure that people know how to keep themselves protected. If only they would pay attention.

—SONIA SINGLETON

□ When asked about her childhood ambition, Sonia responded with her indomitable spirit intact: "My dream was to be a prima ballerina, but my mama told me that in West Palm Beach, where I'm from, there were no black prima ballerinas."

Sonia Singleton died in a Florida hospital on February 19, 1992.

For years Frank Batey waged public warfare with his ex-wife for custody of their son, Brian. He was bisexual; she was a fundamentalist Christian. She charged that Frank had sexually molested Brian (the charges were dismissed in court). In later years, after a judge reverted custody to Frank—a decision that was heralded as a breakthrough for thousands of gay fathers—Brian was kidnapped by his mother.

Eighteen months later, after more legal wranglings, Brian was found and returned to live with his father.

Then, after 13 years of struggle to be with his son, Frank Batey learned that he was HIV-positive. Craig Corbett was Frank's partner in the arduous battle, and his lover of some 13 years.

Brian was about three years old when Frank split up with his ex-wife. Frank discovered that he liked men better than women, and he had been kind of coming out. He had had a few experiences, but they were very minor. I met Frank and fell in love with him. Right after Frank left his wife, she accused him of sexually molesting Brian. She wasn't allowing Frank any contact with Brian. We went to court. She wanted his money, but she didn't want Frank to be able to see him. She cut off all visitation. Finally, the psychologist examined Brian, and Brian said that [the abuse] never happened. So, after a year, they gave Frank regular visitation rights.

When Brian was 11, his mother refused to even let Brian read a letter from Frank. She also cut off all telephone communication between them. Finally, the judge could see that she wasn't going to allow visitation, and that's when we were finally given custody.

But on her first visitation, she kidnapped Brian. She moved out of her apartment and stored all of her furniture and stuff and took off across the country, and they went all through the South, stopping off at these Pentecostal churches that were kind of refuges for them. During this period Frank wrote every social security office in the South and sent flyers and reward posters out to all the hospitals, all the schools, and all the Pentecostal churches that he could think of, thousands of them. After a few months the FBI got involved, and we had a private detective working on it. It turned out that she was living with an elderly lady, a Pentecostal minister. They lived in a house trailer somewhere down in Texas, and she kept Brian out of school. For two years he got no education whatsoever.

Anyway, she turned herself in, and it was a big national news story. But she refused to turn Brian over. Finally, the judge slapped her in jail, but after a couple of weeks she dug Brian out of the woodwork [she was eventually cleared of felony kidnapping charges]. Then, after five foster homes, the courts finally decided to turn Brian over to his dad.

Meanwhile Frank had not been feeling too well, so we both went in and got tested. He tested positive; I was negative. He didn't tell Brian for a very long time. I kept encouraging him to do it, and finally he did. Brian didn't know exactly what being HIV-positive meant. As gently as possible, I explained what the long-term ramifications might be. I said, "There's a chance Dad won't make it."

If Frank's ex-wife had known about his being HIV-positive, she would have taken it back to court. That's one reason Frank didn't want anybody to know about it. But it was becoming quite obvious that he wasn't looking very good. He looked really tired and old and had all the symptoms. Still, he didn't want anybody to know. A lot of our friends didn't even know.

It became public when he died. He had cytomegalovirus in his intestinal tract and bled to death. The phone started ringing, and it rang 3,000 times. I had people from all over the country calling. I couldn't talk at first. I was really broken up. But then I thought that I owed it to Frank to talk about this, and so I started talking to people and did the best I could and tried to be really honest. Most were men calling to thank Frank for what he had done to help them have a relationship with their children. Frank had been one of the first gay fathers in the United States to get custody of his child.

The evening he died, I woke up, and it was all over the news. It was two o'clock in the morning. I looked down the hall and here were five Pentecostals screaming and pounding on Brian's door. They had broken into the house and pushed aside my house guest. They thought that Brian was drugged and locked in a room.

The next day his mother came with the police saying that she wanted to talk to Brian. She got him in the car to go have a hamburger, and they just kept going. They went to San Diego. Finally Brian had a chance to get away, and he ran down to a convenience store and called a friend of mine to pick him up. The next day he petitioned the court that I become his legal guardian.

> *"I loved my father and will miss him terribly. At least
> I have some good memories. This has been my home
> with my father and Craig. He gave a hell of a fight."*
> —**BRIAN BATEY**

Frank wanted me to have custody of Brian more than anything. But he didn't know if that was a possibility, because I was not a natural parent. I wasn't surprised when I got custody of Brian—I was shocked! I was tickled to death. I loved him. I'd known him since he was a baby. He was like my own kid. When he was gone for that week, I was a wreck. I had had a lover and his child in this house, and all of a sudden I had nothing.

How did I get through Frank's illness?

When you've got a kid around who's real active, you're just too busy doing laundry, driving people to school, and running to the doctor. You don't have time to think about that stuff. It's a very difficult thing to go through with a lover. I stayed and took care of Frank. I slept with him every night. I tried to cook everything he liked. I really tried to do things for him, because I knew it was not going to last forever. I'm glad I could do that. It made me happy.

Was it all worth it?

I've spent about a million dollars of my personal funds financing this [child custody] fiasco. I mean, this whole experience was just totally unnecessary. As for taking care of Frank, I have no regrets. We had a nice life together. He never gave up. He never once complained.

It's an amazing thing, the human mind. Even though you may know you're going to die, you don't want to, and you don't think you will. I know. I watched my father die, I watched my mom die, and I watched Frank die. But I don't think any of them thought they were going anyplace.

—CRAIG CORBETT

☐ **Frank Batey died of AIDS on June 16, 1987, the day before his 42nd birthday.**
  As of this writing, Brian Batey, 21, is happily married and living in Missouri. Says his "co-dad," Craig Corbett, "She seems like a really nice girl."

Two days before his death on November 1, 1991, 36-year-old Derrick DeBini wrote a letter to his family and loved ones. It was a letter, says his mother, Shirley, "not only to say good-bye, but a letter of courage for anyone who has a burden to face. It shows that my son had the courage to die. And now we have to have the courage to live."

Shirley DeBini has graciously allowed us to reprint Derrick's letter below.

Three months ago I lay in a hospital bed convinced that I was going to die. AIDS, cancer and pneumonia all seemed to be fighting to claim my life. At that time I felt very terrified that I might die and go to hell, or just not go on at all. But my time had not come. The time since then has been a precious gift in which great healing has occurred. After months of medical treatment, along with months of holistic treatment and months of spiritual work on myself . . . I am free. My lover's remarkable support, a spiritual guide, meditation, several retreats, support from wonderful friends, and a lot of work within my own heart have left me at peace.

For many months my idea of healing was that of curing my body.

253

I gave it my best try, and I am proud of this fact. I was even given several months of relative health and energy at that time. I often expressed my certainty that I could heal my body with my own healing powers. I still believe these healing powers exist, but as my physical health reached a point where optimism about my health would have had to become self-denial, I realized the need to accept my own impending death and physical mortality. I also realized that self-compassion meant feeling in my heart that even death was not a sign of weakness or failure. This seems to be the ultimate factor of self-acceptance. I thank God for it.

All of this did not come easily. I have wept many times. I have gotten angry and confused. But I have learned that the only way out of the pain is through the pain. A hard lesson to learn.

Another thing I have learned is that anytime you think you are absolutely right, you can be sure you're not. "Rightness" is just our trying to prove that someone else is wrong. But we often confuse being right with truth.

In the last year I have installed the data-processing system of a major apparel manufacturer. I have worked to heighten awareness of this insidious disease. I have grown closer than ever to my family, my lover, and my friends. I am very proud and thankful for these things. Most importantly, I have come to accept myself as I am. This is the greatest gift of all, and so my healing has occurred.

Soon my body will be dropping away from me like a cocoon, and my spirit will fly like a butterfly, beautiful and perfect. I don't claim to know where exactly it is that I am going, but my heart tells me that it is filled with light and love. Our time is too short for pettiness, for angry words, for wounded feelings, for crushed souls. An open heart is an infinitely greater blessing than death is a tragedy.

Perhaps the measure of a life is not its length—but its love.

—*DERRICK DeBINI*

Alan Menken and Howard Ashman were close friends, collaborators, and the considerable creative forces responsible for, among other things, the music for the motion pictures *Little Shop of Horrors, The Little Mermaid,* and *Beauty and the Beast.*

On March 14, 1991, at the age of 40, Howard Ashman died of AIDS. He left behind a beloved musical legacy, his family, and Bill, his significant other. He also left behind Alan Menken, who continues to develop their work and pursue their dreams. "We were collaborators; that's more important than being friends," says Alan with a smile. "*And* we were friends. And we were brothers."

To me, an Oscar is small potatoes [compared] to what Howard should have received. Howard won the Oscar for writing the lyrics to the song "Under the Sea" [from *The Little Mermaid*]. He was a brilliant lyricist. But he was also the conceiver of the entire structure of the story, where all the songs would go, and how the whole score would work. Howard was a brilliant director with a brilliant mind. The Oscar was very important to him. I remember sitting in the Oscar party when Howard said to me, "Alan, I want you to know I'm happy. I'm really happy." I said, "Great!" And he said, "Listen, when we get back to New York, we should have a talk." I said, "What about?" He said, "When we get back to New York we'll talk about it." Of course, that was the talk when he told me he had AIDS.

He was always very concerned that the work would stop, that it would interfere with our work if he let people know. But he let me know when he finally had to. That was in early April of 1990. I found out that Howard had been sick for about three years before that.

I hated being told the news. Instantly I was in tears. But it was probably the single most important moment in our relationship. It unburdened him. You don't know the depth of the feelings [we shared]. I mean, collaborators are *partners*.

Over the course of the next year he unburdened himself repeatedly to me about many different things. It was a year of letting go. Still, we had to go on and do a tremendous amount of work with him sick. We had to write all of *Beauty and the Beast* and produce all of it, plus discuss a lot of other projects that we had going on. The work had to get done, and Howard didn't want anyone else but me to know that he was sick. So we had to do a lot of protecting people from knowing. Of course people *did* know, but it was important to him to feel for as long as possible that they didn't.

His life played itself out with a great, bittersweet intensity. There were so many goals that were realized. And yet so many doors were open that he knew he couldn't walk through. That pained him a great deal. He wanted to finish his work. He had completed a lot, but Howard Ashman's goals were *enormous*. And they were the kind of goals that most people will never even dream of, much less pursue. Howard, had he lived, would have been one of the major creative artists in American history. I have no doubt about that. And he knew it. And he was resigned to the parade passing him by.

How did I get through his illness and death?

By letting it be OK that he was sick. By letting it be OK that AIDS exists. By not railing against it and fighting it and trying to figure out *why?* I would say to myself, Well, Howard's relatively healthy. And when I didn't have that anymore, I said, Well, Howard's alive. And when he died, my life went into a flurry of activity. I cried, but I was so busy that I was able to kind of keep pushing along. And then when the Golden Globe nominations for *Beauty and the Beast* happened, I just sank into a very deep depression. I think that the mourning process has really stretched itself out for me. I'm still very much in it.

When Howard first told me that he was sick, right after the Oscars, he said to me, "I feel good telling you now because I know that you'll be taken care of." Howard was like that. That's something that I'll always remember.

Howard is in everything I do. When I wrote the score for *Beauty and the Beast,* there was a theme called "Transformation," and it starts with this very soft cello line that's playing "Beauty and the Beast." I always think of Howard when I hear that. That, to me, is my little funeral march for Howard Ashman. Today he is the standard by which I judge everything I do.

—*ALAN MENKEN*

❏   ❏

Roxy and Vincent Ventola had been friends, lovers, and
writing partners since 1983. They married in 1984, and
there was only one thing missing from their idyllic
romance.

For the next six years Roxy and Vincent invested their
love, time, and money, not to mention a considerable
amount of physical and emotional pain, in a single,
shared dream: the dream of having the baby they
desperately wanted.

She was a miracle child. It was major experimental surgery that I
had. This was our last shot. This was all the money we had left.
When I went into the hospital for the surgery, the general anesthetic
made me nauseous, and I threw up the estrogen. The next day the
doctor told me that I didn't have anywhere near the estrogen levels
needed to have a baby implant, and they told me that I was not
going to be pregnant. But I knew that I *was*. I don't know how to
explain it. So they actually rewrote their medical knowledge. It was
a rough pregnancy in a certain way, because I had twins. On Christmas Eve I miscarried one of them, and I had to stay in bed for five
months and take progesterone shots, which were really painful, so

that I didn't miscarry the other one. But I did it gratefully, because we were just so thrilled to have this dream coming true.

Miranda was born on August 5, 1989, and she was perfectly healthy. I had all of the best doctors, she was a great baby, and we learned how to be good parents. It was December 22, and I thought I was just being a nervous mom. Miranda seemed a little less energetic. She seemed to be sleeping a little more than usual. I said to Vinnie, "Look, this is our first Christmas as a family. I'm nervous. I don't want anything to blow it. She's probably getting a cold. Let's take her to the pediatrician, just to calm me down so we can enjoy this holiday."

So we went to the pediatrician, he examined her, and everything was fine. But as I was dressing her to leave, she turned blue. We went to the hospital, she had a chest X ray, and it was determined that she had viral pneumonia, which was epidemic in children and babies at that time. She was admitted into the hospital on oxygen, and they said, "Don't worry, this will take a few days. We have this treatment."

She went into the intensive-care unit, and she didn't get better. They did everything, and finally they had her on 100 percent oxygen. Then both of her lungs collapsed at the same time, and she went on a respirator. I'll never forget it. It was on New Year's Eve, and they said, "She can't stay on the respirator anymore or else she'll never be able to come off it." You can only be on 100 percent oxygen for a certain amount of time. The only other option was to use an ECMO [extracorporeal membrane oxygenation] machine, a heart-and-lung bypass machine, so that they could close down her lungs and give them a chance to heal. They would take her blood out through her carotid artery, oxygenate it, and put it back in. The only problem was that there were only two such machines in all of California. Miraculously one of them opened up. I asked the doctor,

"What would you do if it was your child?" And he said, "There is a great risk of putting her on this machine, but you have no choice."

She was transferred to UCLA a little bit before midnight. I'll never forget it. Vinnie and I were following the ambulance, riding through the streets of Westwood. All the college kids were coming out of their fraternity houses and their sorority houses and celebrating 1990.

Anyway, we met with the surgeons and they put her on the machine. We were very frightened, because there was a very high risk of brain damage and death. She was on the machine for seven days, and it was horrible. Truly horrible. It was like a Frankenstein movie. All these teams of doctors kept examining her. I didn't know who they all were, and they kept conferring. And every day they kept telling us that they had ruled out this horrible disease and that horrible disease. But they couldn't find out why she wasn't getting any better.

The day they took her off the machine, we had about 20 minutes to celebrate. They did a brain scan on her and everything, and it looked like a real miracle had happened. Then the immunologists and the infectious-disease doctors stood in the hallway outside of pediatric intensive care and told us that Miranda had pneumocystis. I couldn't understand. What is pneumocystis, you know? And then they told us she had AIDS.

It's as if I had gone from one life and was put on a space shuttle and taken to another world. You have to understand that for us, when we had our child, we felt that our dreams were finally being realized. We were so honored to be parents. Most people take that privilege for granted. I don't think they understand the gift that they have. All we filled ourselves with was how we wanted to provide the most secure atmosphere for our child. We had a television show "go" and we sold a screenplay while I was pregnant. And it was like, all of a sudden, everything we had worked so hard for, emotionally and physically, was happening. We were reaping the rewards of years and years of struggle. Then we were given the diagnosis, and I felt like I was being thrown out of paradise.

They told us when we took her home from the hospital that she wouldn't live more than two months, because no child had ever survived pneumocystis longer than two months. But she astounded everyone and developed normally. She never even had a cold or an infection. She talked, she walked, she gained weight.

The virus was totally dormant in her system because of the AZT she was taking. What happened, though, was that she developed a white-cell anemia, a side effect of the AZT. We had to keep lowering her dosage, and the doctor kept saying, "Well, there is this new drug that could offset the anemia, but we haven't gotten it yet." Finally, in the fall, the doctor told us that we had to put her on DDI. So we did, but it didn't absorb into her body. We didn't know it then, but she was getting gradually weaker. Well, the virus attacked her central nervous system. She got encephalopathy. It took away her gross motor skills, her language skills, and some of her fine motor skills. You know, her hands and stuff.

In December we pulled strings and got the drug company to release this new drug, a growth-stimulating hormone, under the Compassionate Children's Act. So we put her back on the AZT, and the virus went dormant again. But the damage had already been done. We put her on steroids, because there was a theory that they could clean the virus out of her brain. And she did make some progress, but she never crawled again.

A few days after we found out that Miranda had AIDS, Vinnie and I both got tested. Both tests came back HIV-positive. In April of 1991 Vinnie had a cancerous tumor in his hip. It wasn't lymphoma; it wasn't an AIDS-related tumor; that's the irony. It was a very treatable kind of tumor with a 90 percent success rate—in a person with a normal immune system. He went in for radiation treatments, and they knocked his immune system down. It was regular pneumonia, and he still wasn't diagnosed with AIDS. He lost a lot of weight and started to physically falter. We got him back into the hospital, and they discovered some spots on his lungs. Then they gave him chemotherapy. He was doing OK with the first two treatments, but the third treatment almost killed him. He was horribly weak and nauseous. He lost all of his hair, and then he got CMV. The doctors thought he would die right then. He didn't. He fought. That was in the summer, around July.

Vinnie took AZT, but that gave him a terrible red-cell anemia, and he did something else for a while, and then the doctor switched him to DDI. But he got terrible neuropathy in his feet from it, and he just stopped taking it. He didn't want to take anything else. He was on so much stuff. They put him on TPN [total parental nutrition], which is like a liquid gold food. One day they took him off it too fast, and he had a grand-mal seizure. It was horrible. I rushed him to the hospital. With both Vinnie and Miranda it was almost overwhelming.

When he got back home, I said to him, "I'm going to get all this stuff out of you and I'm going to cook!" And so I became this gourmet cook and made Vinnie gain 24 pounds. Even Miranda gained a pound, and I thought maybe we could stop all this [deterioration].

The doctors were all amazed by Vinnie's recovery. He was quite energetic. He was driving himself to doctors' appointments, doing errands. Then one day he had a sinus infection. He was always getting little sinus infections. And I said to him, "I want you to go to the doctor immediately, because you cannot afford to have an infection in your system." So he called the doctor and made an appointment for Thursday. On the Tuesday before that, Vinnie insisted on taking Miranda to her doctor at UCLA without me. He took a girlfriend of mine to help him. I remember it took them a long, long time to come home, and when they did, he looked horrible, and my girlfriend was acting weird. I said, "What's wrong? Is this bad news?" And he said "No." What he didn't tell me, and what I found out later, was that they had told him Miranda was dying. He didn't want to tell me because he wanted to protect me.

I think it was then that Vinnie decided to die too. He loved Miranda more than he loved anything ever in his life, and I don't think he could bear to see her die. We both went through a lot of guilt for giving our child this disease, even though we didn't know it. But it's a disease you give to people you love. And to give it to your child is almost unbearable to take.

On Thursday Vinnie went to his appointment at the hospital and decided to stay there. He packed a bag and didn't tell me. When we talked on the phone, I was angry. But I talked to his doctor on Saturday who said, "Well, it was just an infection from the sinuses that got into his bloodstream. He is on IV penicillin and will be home on Monday."

Then, in the middle of that Saturday night, at four in the morning, I got a call from the hospital. The nurse said, "Your husband has taken a terrible downturn." I said, "What about my baby?" She said, "If you have to, stay with the baby. But I really think you've got to come. He won't take any drugs until he talks to you." So I got somebody to watch Miranda. She was crying. She knew something was wrong. She didn't want me to leave. It was so hard for me to leave her then in the middle of the night to go to him. I didn't know where to be.

My girlfriend and I drove to the hospital in Sherman Oaks, and when we got there, he was still hanging on. I had my friend call another friend and get on the telephone to his parents in New Jersey, my parents in Brooklyn, and my brother in San Francisco, and all of our friends. I knew that Vinnie was going to die. I thought, We have to help him through this. We've got to make this a happy occasion for him so that he can die bravely, with dignity, and surrounded by love. Friends came in, and we told him funny stories. Vinnie was a very funny guy. He had a great sense of humor. I told him funny stories. I told him our love story and all the great times I had with him and how much we all loved him. I told him about the wonderful place he was going to where there would be no more suffering, because I believe in God and in an afterlife. Then we had a party, and our doctor, on his only day off, stayed there all day. At a certain point we decided to put Vinnie on a morphine drip, because he was in pain and so he wouldn't have to suffer. But he was aware and conscious until the end. For a few hours before the end he couldn't talk anymore. It was hard for him to breathe. His breaths became longer and longer. I said to him, "Why are you hanging on, sweetheart? For once in your life, put yourself first now. Why are you just hanging here?" And he pointed at me. I said, "You don't have to be afraid to leave me. I promise you, I'll take care of myself and our baby. I'll handle this, I promise you. And I'll see you again. Someday. And I've always loved you. You're the best thing that's ever happened in my life. I have not one regret. I would follow you to hell and back. And to heaven." He cried a tear. One tear. And he motioned for me to kiss him and hold him. He closed his eyes. And he smiled. I feel like he saw the angels. And he died.

It was November 17, 1991. Miranda died six days later.

How have I gotten through this?

I don't belong to any religion, but, faith, that's how I've gotten through this. Faith in God. Faith that I will see my child and my husband again. Faith that they are happy now and in healthy bodies.

Faith that they are in peace. I believe the human spirit is eternal. I really, truly believe that this is not just a wrap, you know?

I've also decided that this isn't a cruel thing. This is a gift that God has given me to do good. I've decided to try to make a difference and honor the 130,000 people in this country who have bravely died in this health war. And to try to wake up the one million people who are probably infected right now and don't even know it, and the countless others who maybe could save their own lives. I want to try to change attitudes, because the silence, the lack of compassion, and the bigotry is worse than the disease itself. I want to talk to people who think this disease can't touch them. Basically I'm trying to wake up the heterosexual community.

This disease just doesn't knock on the door like Santa Claus and ask if you've been good or bad. It takes just one encounter to get this disease. Sex and death have come together in one disease and pushed every bigoted button in this country. It's insane to me. So if they want to treat me like a leper, then I want to be on the island of Molokai with all my friends and doctors. But until they give me that island, I'm going to be in their face, in a pleasant way, in any way that I can, to communicate and change attitudes. It's bad enough we have a death sentence, but God damn it, they're not going to make my life worse, or anyone's life worse, while I'm alive. I'm going to fight that.

What would I say to others?

One thing I've learned when dealing with people who are uninvolved or bigoted: I would never give them the answer to the question, *"How* did you get this disease?" It seems to be their first question. And I don't think that question deserves an answer. I don't know *how* I got it, and if I did, it's nobody's business. They just want to pass judgment. We don't deserve to have our lives scrutinized by people who are more fortunate than we are. So I would suggest that you never tell how you got it, that you make people feel uncomfortable when they ask such a rude question.

Second, I would say to tell people that you are infected. For a year Vinnie and I were in the closet. When we started telling people, the reaction we got from heterosexuals was horrible. They all dropped us. It was very painful. So we went back into the closet, but that was a different kind of hell. You are living with a wall around you, in isolation. And you're not letting in the people who really could be there to love and help you. So I would say, just take the plunge and tell everybody. Make it a test. The true friends and the true family members who love you will be there, and they'll be there stronger than ever. Get rid of the dead wood.

The third thing I would say is to develop a faith in something higher than yourself, whatever that is. It helps a lot. This isn't the end. It would be too cruel if this was the only part of life.

I would also say to get rid of the blame. That's going to be your biggest struggle. Don't blame yourself, don't blame others, don't blame the world. Get rid of the phase of anger that you are going to be through, because you're just poisoning your own quality of life with it. Use those feelings constructively. Know that you've done nothing wrong. We don't even execute serial killers in this country. Don't buy into anybody else's trip. Let your life prove their attitudes to be a lie. Let your life be so wonderful, so full of love and joy and happiness and good feelings that the light is going to blind those in the dark.

—ROXY VENTOLA

☐ Vincent Ventola was 44 years old at the time of his death. Miranda Rose was two years and three months. As of this writing Roxy Ventola, 44, the wife and mother they left behind, is an AIDS educator. She is still relatively healthy and still emanating love and light.

When asked what she missed most, Roxy responded, "Holding my baby. Sitting down on the couch next to Vinnie."

David Andrew Deyo was born in Oak Park, Illinois. He moved to Washington, D.C., in 1975 and studied at Gallaudet University, where he earned two master's degrees—one in audiology in 1977 and the other in educational technology in 1987. While at Gallaudet, David was twice named a presidential scholar and was active with the American Speech and Hearing Association and the D.C. Speech and Hearing Association. He was also working on his dissertation, "AIDS Policies and Education in Schools and Programs for the Deaf," with hopes of completing a Ph.D. in supervision and management in May 1992.

David Deyo was diagnosed HIV-positive in 1984. Still, he persisted with his work and studies until his death on November 25, 1991. He was 39 years old.

On the following pages David is remembered by his mother, Virginia, and by his own words, taken from his journal, which Virginia has graciously allowed us to reprint.

David ended up in the hospital on Easter Sunday of 1989 with pneumonia. Somehow he got through that. David used to say that there were three things that helped him get through this disease: to have a positive attitude, to continue to exercise, and to have goals. Even if it was a small goal. This is his journal entry for Thanksgiving 1989:

> Earl and I decided to have a big Thanksgiving-day celebration this year. We had a lot to be thankful for. Both of us are still alive and in relatively good health. We have a beautiful home and supportive friends and family. Why not be thankful?
>
> Earl took the responsibility for the turkeys and ham, so I decided to make my traditional pickled peaches and cranberry relish, but somehow it didn't seem enough. So during the six to seven weeks before Thanksgiving I embarked on a major home-improvement project. I decided that I was tired of all off-white walls and that I would paint as many rooms as I could before Thanksgiving came. Not a small task considering I was often in a weakened condition and our house has cathedral ceilings and some 12-foot walls. . . .
>
> There was more to it than the simple act of painting. I experienced a wonderful sense of enjoyment and fulfillment from the process. Not only did I make the environment more beautiful and comfortable, I proved something to myself and to those around me. This was my project. I conceived it, I planned it, and (in spite of my illness) I executed it. I could have just sat around the house looking at the off-white walls and wondering what it might be like to add a little color. . . .
>
> I did it! I took my time, I worked some days and rested on others. And I accomplished what seemed like a herculean task and did it in time for our Thanksgiving celebration!

Of course his big goal was to get his Ph.D. That's what he wanted most. He had done everything for the program, except finishing the dissertation. He'd gathered all the material for it, it was all in the computer, and he was going to start to write it. And then he got so ill last fall that he couldn't do it. As I understand it, a few of his friends have gotten together and have formed a study group. They are going to try and write this material for him, present it, and get it published. They are hoping to get him his Ph.D. I just can't believe they are doing this for him.

David lived up there in Maryland. I live in Florida. We communicated through letters and phone calls. David was always very optimistic, and that helped me a great deal. He was cheerful, and he never moaned and groaned. He was just so good about it. That helped so much. You know that there is a deep problem there, but his spirit was so wonderful and so inspiring that you can't break up, and you can't let down. If he's not going to let down, you're not either, you know? He had such a positive attitude.

> *"Each new day gives us a chance to make a fresh start. Like all those first days of school that we faced as children each September. If we're armed with our pencil box, our new set of crayons, and our peanut-butter sandwich, we can face anything!"*
>
> **—DAVID DEYO**
> loosely interpreted from
> the words of his longtime companion,
> the Reverend Earl Tallman

Strangely enough, David got active AIDS before Earl, and then Earl was his caregiver. Somewhere along the line, Earl became seriously ill with AIDS, and David, even though he too was sick, became Earl's caregiver. He was with Earl to the end. In his journal he wrote:

270

The month of October has been particularly hard on me. As I was in the midst of my comprehensive exams for my Ph.D. program, I lost my father to cancer. Now I'm sitting here watching Earl in bed as he slips further and further away from me. Yesterday he could talk a little; today he can't. Yesterday he could shake his head for yes and no. Today he can't. The pain is getting unbearable. For him and for me. Earl is now taking morphine. What am I supposed to take? How do you soothe a broken heart? A broken soul? You watch the person you love slowly slip away into unconsciousness with nothing that you can do.

So as I sit here and watch him sleep tonight, the best I can do is to say good-bye. Lovingly, tearfully, but not with regret. . . . Good-bye, my dear friend, my best friend. I will miss you every day.

My mother passed away in May of 1990. She was 97. In October of that year my husband died of lung cancer. Then, 11 days after his father died, David's dear friend Earl Tallman died. What a burden this poor boy had. We didn't have the memorial service for my husband as soon as we might have, because David was going through the very worst part of everything with Earl, who was on his deathbed. And he said, "Mother, I can't come. I can't leave Earl." I said, "Well, there isn't going to be any memorial service unless all of you boys are here. So we just won't have it the first week." So after Earl's death, David was free to come to the memorial service for his father. It was a dreadful, dreadful time for this poor boy.

Actually, I thought, the Lord has been good to me. He took my mother first so that I could concentrate on the illness of my husband. Then the Lord took my husband, and He took him quickly when it finally did come. In six days he was gone. Then I could turn my attention to David, if he needed me.

After the pneumonia, David got meningitis. He had a lot of anemia, he got staph infections, both of his lungs collapsed, he lost over 30 pounds. He was all skin and bones. Finally, neurological disorders toward the end really debilitated him. They made it very difficult for him to talk. There was such great weakness that he couldn't really do much of anything.

At the time his lungs collapsed, I didn't go to him. As soon as he got out of the hospital, I stayed with him at home while he was recuperating. I never could have done that if my husband had still been living. I would have had to stay with my husband. So I just felt like the Lord took care of me in that way.

I was also fortunate in another way. David called and said that he needed me. I arrived on Sunday, and he was gone on Monday at noon. I was his caregiver for the last night of his life. He had his faculties, his mind, to the end. But when he would get weak, he wouldn't say much. There wasn't any real communication with him on that last visit. I regret very much that I didn't get there a little bit before that, when he was still talking, but he wanted it that way. He wanted to remain independent as long as he could. Looking back on it now, I think he was really trying to spare me. I think he thought it would be easier on me not to come into the picture until the very end. His friends had been taking such marvelous care of him. They had people there constantly with him, sleeping overnight, tending to his needs.

How have I gotten through this?

I have gotten so much comfort out of his friends, I can't tell you. It was just the most wonderful revelation to me when I was there after he died and I saw how supportive these young people were, and how much they cared for my boy. Of course I cared for him too, but I always felt that maybe I was prejudiced in thinking that he was such a wonderful person. But when I realized that all

these other people felt the same way I did, that was the most wonderful thing to me.

—*VIRGINIA DEYO*

☐ At one point during their big Thanksgiving celebration
of 1989, David Deyo and Earl Tallman summoned all of
their friends into the living room, and David lifted his
glass for a special toast. He then gave an impromptu
speech, which he later printed in his journal, that
seems particularly poignant and relevant and a perfect
way to close these pages.

*"Today is Thanksgiving. There are a few things that I
feel a need to say, and this seems to be a good time to
do it.*

*As most of you know, this past year has not been
an easy one for me. . . . actually, for both Earl and
me. I have had some serious health problems. Last
spring when I was really sick and in the hospital, I
had serious doubts that I would still be alive to
celebrate the holidays this year. Earl has had his
doubts too. He told me a few weeks ago that the
reason we're having a big celebration this year is
because this might be our last Thanksgiving together.
But I refuse to accept that! I plan to be here for
Thanksgiving next year! (Applause breaks out at this
point.) And I hope that you all plan to be here too.*

*So today I would like to propose a toast to all of
you. This is a two-part toast. The first part is to*

friends. You've all been there for me this past year, and it's really meant a lot to me (I'm close to tears).

I hope that you'll continue to be there for me next year, and the next, and the next. . . . The second part of my toast is to life. Through this illness I've discovered how beautiful life is (more tears now). On my good days and on my bad days. It doesn't matter. Each day it's just wonderful to be here and to be alive.

So if you'll all raise your glasses with me, I'd like to propose a toast—to life!"

—FROM DAVID DEYO'S JOURNAL

SOURCES

Voices That Care is almost completely based on interviews conducted by the author. A few quotes, however, were derived from other sources. Those sources, and the specific quotes reprinted, are credited below. All but three of the celebrity entries were derived from original interviews for this book. The statements by Elizabeth Taylor, Jerry Brown, and Phil Donahue were previously released and are reprinted herein with permission.

JUNE KENNEY

Following are the first words of the quotations from the *Los Angeles Times*, August 22, 1991:

Following are the first words of the quotations from *Yankee*, July 1991:

STEPHEN PIETERS

Following are the first words of the quotations from "AIDS Alumnus" by Neal Turnage, published in *Optimist* (Winter 1991–92):

DR. DON HAGAN

Following are the first words of the quotations from the *Los Angeles Times*, September 17, 1991:

BUDDY MONTGOMERY

Following are the first words of the quotations from the *Bay Area Reporter*, August 29, 1991:

CAROL LYNN PEARSON

Following are the first words of the quotations from *Good-bye, I Love You* (Random House 1986) by Carol Lynn Pearson:

JUDGE RAND SCHRADER

Following are the first words of the quotations from the *Los Angeles Times*, November 25, 1991:

CRAIG CORBETT

Following are the first words of the quotation from the *Los Angeles Times*, June 27, 1987: